Prentice-Hall International, Inc., *London*
Prentice-Hall of Australia, Pty, Ltd., *Sydney*
Prentice-Hall Canada, Inc., *Toronto*
Prentice-Hall of India Private Ltd., *New Delhi*
Prentice-Hall of Japan, Inc. *Tokyo*
Prentice-Hall of Southeast Asia Pte. Ltd., *Singapore*
Whitehall Books, Ltd., *Wellington, New Zealand*
Editora Prentice-Hall do Brasil Ltda., *Rio de Janeiro*
Prentice-Hall Hispanoamericana, S.A., *Mexico*

This book is a reference work based on research by the author. The opinions expressed herein are not necessarily those of or endorsed by the publisher. The directions stated in this book are in no way to be considered as a substitute for consultation with a duly licensed doctor.

Library of Congress Cataloging-in-Publication Data

Daro, August F.
Dr. Daro's Nutrition prescriptions for your common health problems.

Includes index.
1. Diet therapy. 2. Nutrition. 3. Medicine, Popular. I. Banke, Walter J. II. Title. III. Title: Nutrition prescriptions for your common health problems. [DNLM: 1. Diet Therapy—popular works. 2. Nutrition—popular works. WB 400 D224n]
RM216.D26 1986 615.8'54 85-30091

ISBN 0-13-216300-4

Printed in the United States of America

"Dear Dr. Daro..."

"Please let me know what vitamin and how much I can take for poor circulation of the blood.

"When I lift my hands to comb my hair or sleep on one side or the other my fingers and hands fall asleep. I have had this two years and I am 48 years old."

"Your work in the field of nutrition was recently featured in a (Chicago) Tribune article...it impressed me! I have glomerulonephritis and have had it since the birth of our daughter three years ago. Currently I am taking diuretics and have been treated in the past with prednisone and indocin; both of which have had little or no success. My doctor has had me on a low sodium, high protein, low cholesterol diet and like most doctors does not advise vitamins.

"Could you please help me?"

"I just finished reading your article in *Prevention* magazine and was greatly impressed.

"I've spent literally hundreds of dollars going from doctors to specialists to chiropractors having all kinds of x-rays, tests, etc., all to no avail.

"I've been suffering for 21 years with constant headaches. I have one all day long and even wake up with one. I'm told I have some cervical arthritis and mainly tension headaches."

"I am enormously interested in the article about you done by *Prevention* magazine.

"Because I am confused about all the published material on supplements, I was wondering if you could refer me to a doctor here...who is as knowledgeable as you are...I don't want to prescribe for myself but have not been able to find an M.D. who specializes in nutrition in this city (New York, New York) and would be more than grateful for the information."

"Our youngest son has hypoglycemia. He is hyperactive. He has a short attention span. He is disruptive in class.

"...Our son's pediatrician does not believe in hypoglycemia, nutrition, vitamins, etc. We had him tested by another doctor who confirmed that he had hypoglycemia.

"Can you provide me with the name of a doctor (or a list of doctors) that will treat my son properly for this problem."

The preceding represent a few of the very large number of letters that I received in response to articles that appeared about me in *Prevention* and *Bestways* magazines and, also, in the *Chicago Tribune*. Little did I guess when I agreed to the interviews that there was such a pent-up interest in, and demand for, information on nutritional therapy. People seem to be looking for alternatives to conventional medical therapy. This interest and demand has stimulated the growth of health food, vitamin stores and, also, the proliferation of foods that are identified as containing all natural ingredients with no preservatives. I am gratified to see this occurring. If we can improve the health and well-being of people by improving their diet rather than through heroic and dramatic surgical and medical therapies, perhaps we can even start to lower the cost of medical care.

People from all parts of the country requested office appointments after my article appeared. I was amazed that so many people were willing to spend hundreds of dollars on transportation, lodging, and meals for the sole purpose of consulting with a doctor with an interest and background in nutritional therapy. The explanation, of course, is that these people were not able to find medical doctors in their own communities who could counsel them from the nutritional point of view.

As it was, I was able to see only some of the people who contacted me. Unfortunately, I'm afraid that there were many whose letters and calls I was not able to answer or acknowledge. It was simply physically impossible for me to do so and, in addition, I have been reducing my medical practice time. At the present time, I see patients only a few days a week. However, what the outpouring of mail and calls did do was stimulate my thinking that, perhaps, I might be able to help on a broader scale by setting down some of my experiences with nutrition as a very important and simple route to improve health.

What This Book Will Do for You

As you read my experiences and comments, I am confident that you will come away more aware that changes in your eating habits and vitamin-mineral supplementation can bring improvements in your physical health, mental attitude, and work output. The patients I have helped are just like you but perhaps didn't realize how their health was affected when they relied on junk foods, missed meals, and generally paid no attention to what science proves we need in the way of vitamins, minerals, and other nutrients. It's true that you can't control what heredity gives you in the way of your body and physiological systems but you can improve the functioning of what you have. Even some hereditary diseases can be helped through diet alteration.

I hope that this book will make you believe that if you treat your body well through sound nutritional practices, it will give you 70, 80, or even more years of faithful service. No matter what your age, you can make improvements in the way you feel. You might compare this book to the car owner's manual provided when you buy a new car. What I am giving you here is a body owner's manual for health maintenance and improvement.

At the outset I want to mention that the information presented is not based on controlled, scientific studies. What I have to say is what I have learned from treating patients with a variety of complaints and illnesses and the results achieved using nutritional ideas. For example, there is the female patient who was advised to have a coronary bypass operation. Instead, she asked me to work out a nutritional approach and we were able to bypass the bypass. A man, 85 years old, suffered from psoriasis, had seen dozens of specialists, and found no permanent relief. I was able to provide him with the first, long-term relief he had ever had. Then, there was the medical colleague I convinced to start taking a vitamin that helped change him from a weary physician making his hospital rounds to an energetic individual. His wife thanked me profusely for the transformation when I encountered the couple on a trip to Rome.

Over and over again, the people writing to me asked for the names of medical doctors to whom they could turn for assistance and who have experience using nutrition as a method of treatment. Physicians, unfortunately, with this interest or background are few in number. However, medical care is undergoing a revolution in the country and more emphasis is being placed on the preventive care that really lies at the core of nutritional therapy. As a result of the new directions medicine is taking, I expect medical doctors with competence in the field of nutritional therapy to grow in numbers. In addition, the increase in health-maintenance organizations has a positive effect because the groups place emphasis on the individual being responsible for his or her well-being with a key point being attention to diet.

As a consumer of health care, you can help the growth and advancement of nutritional therapy. People do get what they ask for and as more and more people demand doctors with knowledge of nutritional concepts, the medical establishment will deliver practitioners who are trained in this field. Equally important is the fact that more research is needed to explain the roles of vitamins, minerals, amino acids, enzymes, and other nutrients in assisting the body to function as optimally as possible.

Research Brings New Solutions to Your Health Problems

Continuing research brings new knowledge and answers involving the importance of nutritional factors. At a recent meeting of the American Heart Association, a Cornell University researcher reported that many people with moderately high blood pressure could probably control it by taking an appropriate mineral supplement. He said that one-third to one-half of the population is salt sensitive, meaning that they develop an elevated blood pressure when they consume the amount of salt eaten by the average American. This, in turn, causes a loss of calcium. He further suggested that it might be easier to add more calcium to the diet than reduce salt intake and that mineral balance might be achieved easier this way.

Through sound nutritional choices, I believe that your body's immune system is helped to defend against infection and the other factors that our environment inflicts on us, such as water and air pollution, noise, extremes of cold and heat, and stresses of an interpersonal nature. Medical studies are tending to confirm that nutritional choices are important in helping the body ward off disease. Rather recently, it has been suggested that eating certain vegetables, cutting down on fat consumption, and eating more whole-grain foods can form a line of defense against cancer. And, as an obstetrician-gynecologist, one area that I cannot neglect mentioning is that the health of future generations depends on how well we take care of our individual reproductive systems, which is tied to the general health of our bodies. Pregnant women who eat fattening foods, smoke, drink alcohol, or use drugs pose a grave danger not only to their own bodies but, obviously, to the developing embryo. Going back a step, women who want to have babies and who follow this life style and eating habits are similarly inviting problems. The same applies to men. If you wish to become a parent, give the unborn child the benefit of your body being in as sound a physical state as possible. Pregnant women who eat soundly and provide their bodies with supplementation with vitamins and minerals stand an excellent chance of bringing into the world healthy and well-developed babies.

As you read the following pages, you will gain new insight and, hopefully, enthusiasm and motivation to start or further your quest for good health and wellness through the nutritional approach. Until such time that scientists discover the all-purpose, health-producing-and-maintaining pill or nutrient factor, you and I will have to rely on existing foods. Since we have a profusion of food choices I want you to be convinced that by making the correct choices you can and will bring yourself new health and well-being.

As you'll see when you read my book, I have helped a number of patients with this approach and I am sure that you can use it to help yourself, too. And, I want to add that the correct food choices will not cost you anymore—financially or physically—than the incorrect ones.

Contents

Dr. Daro's Guide to Health-Promoting Nutrients

Chapter 1

My Early Nutritional Discoveries

Before describing specific medical conditions and how I treat them, I thought I might share with you some aspects of my background. While my "conversion" to a nutrition-oriented physician came late in my practice, there were incidents and cases very early that were shaping my thinking and beliefs. It did not happen that one day I decided to look into the eating habits of my patients to see if there was a nutrition problem as a cause for a medical condition. My emphasis on nutritional therapy happened gradually. I believe that as you read the anecdotes, you will gain insight into your nutritional status. Read along and think back to how some changes in your diet, perhaps, have made an improvement in your health. If that has not occurred, read the anecdotes and analyze how you might alter your diet to achieve a new level of wellness.

We are not born with a health food consciousness or attitude. It takes time and effort, even some wrong turns in the road, to become aware of correct eating habits and nutritional supplementation and their impact on health. What I want to accomplish here is to raise your level of health consciousness as you follow along with my awakening.

How My Early Training Opened My Eyes to the Vital Connection between Nutrition and Health

In 1925, I graduated from the Chicago Medical School, University of Health Sciences (that may give you some indication of how old I am). My internship was served at the Illinois

Masonic Hospital and my residency at the Chicago Lying-In Hospital.

After my residency, I set my sights on obtaining an appointment at the Cook County Hospital. In a single day at this institution, a physician can see, diagnose, and treat scores of medical conditions and ailments that were formerly just dry topics in the medical texts. Service at Cook is a concentrated learning experience that few physicians who have been through it will forget. While appointments to Cook County were difficult to obtain, luck was with me the day I was interviewed by Dr. Karl Meyer, one of Chicago's most illustrious surgeons and, at the time, Chief Medical Officer and Superintendent of the hospital. Something about my enthusiasm must have impressed him because I obtained an assignment in one of the obstetric clinics at the hospital.

The practice of medicine really began in earnest for me at Cook County Hospital where we would see up to 150 pregnant women in a single Wednesday afternoon. As I look back, I believe my nutritional orientation was stimulated when taking medical histories of these patients and seeing a pattern of poor eating habits and low nutritional intake emerging. It was increasingly apparent that these particular patients did not need a prescription drug for their medical problems as much as they needed guidance on what to eat and what supplementation was required.

I continued to work at the clinic for some 20 additional years just to continue to learn and increase my medical knowledge. I was simultaneously building my own private practice, and in working at Cook County, I was exchanging my time for a most concentrated postgraduate education. We were not paid at Cook, but the chance to cope with a broad spectrum of medical and obstetrical cases more than compensated for this. And, it was during this period that I first started to document the importance of nutrition and its influence in health and disease.

In addition to my work at the obstetric clinic, I also performed examinations of patients in the prenatal clinic at Cook County Hospital. While I was not formally placing emphasis on nutrition at this stage of my medical practice, I must have been subconsciously storing information that led many years later to a lot of the conclusions I now share with an increasing number of physicians and other medical practitioners.

My First Nutritional Discovery

On their first visit to the prenatal clinic, patients always received a general physical examination that included an examination of the mouth. In examining the teeth I was struck by the fact that there seemed to be two distinct classes or groups. One group had beautiful noncarious teeth and healthy gums. The second group, on the other hand, had many bad and decaying teeth and swollen and infected gums. I was intrigued by these findings and began a little research project. I carefully questioned these patients and learned that a difference in the type of food eaten and the manner of preparation accounted for my observations. The group with the healthy teeth and gums ate plenty of fresh fruit and vegetables and drank large quantities of milk. The group with the bad teeth relied on starch foods, including cakes, cookies, and pies—in short, food with little nutritional value. However, this finding was, of course, not surprising. What did surprise me was that I found that the group with the bad teeth also reported eating plenty of vegetables. However, when I inquired as to how long the vegetables were cooked, the answer invariably would be, "...until they are soft."

How People Unknowingly Destroy Valuable Nutrients

By overheating and overcooking, this group of patients was effectively destroying most of the vitamin and mineral content of the vegetables they ate. The water-soluble vitamins were leached out of the vegetables and into the water that was then, undoubtedly, dumped into the sink. It would have been far better had they dumped the vegetables at this point and drank the cooking water.

This lesson has become a cornerstone of my recommendations when I talk diet with patients. Very simply stated—

don't overcook–don't boil too long. Many of you reading this will, perhaps, say to yourselves that this is not a very remarkable piece of nutritional advice. But, you would be surprised to learn, just as I am after 58 years of medical practice, that a lot of people still do not know or understand that prolonged heating destroys what is valuable in food.

First Step to Good Health

Even worse from the standpoint of good health is the fact that so many people eat so little in the way of fresh fruit and vegetables. I understand, of course, that not all people can eat or will like all foods. People can and will be allergic to certain foods. Nevertheless, in the United States there is a sufficient variety of food, so that an individual can select at least one or two items to try and eat from the important food groups of fish, meat, fruits, vegetables, milk, eggs, cheese, and cereals. And, there are hundreds of cookbooks available with recipes for preparing these foods in different and appetizing ways. Maybe your mother did prepare spinach in a way that did not please your palate. But that should not be the end of your effort to find a way to prepare spinach that will be appetizing to you. A little seasoning or a dab of dressing may be all that is needed to turn some disliked but nutritionally important food into one of your favorite dishes.

Always Better—Fresh Fruits and Vegetables

You may wonder why I have spent so much space here discussing the importance of the basic food groups. I continue to be surprised at the number of people who come to me with only the foggiest idea of balanced eating habits. Perhaps one of the chief adversaries to good eating habits are the fast-food restaurants. In these establishments, until the recent addition of salad bars, it has been difficult to see a vegetable anywhere on the menu—hamburgers, milk shakes, pies, and cookies, yes. Broccoli, zucchini, squash, string beans, or cauliflower—no. I am sure that there are studies and evidence that demonstrate that these meals provide some of the important minerals and vitamins. In addition, frozen entrees and convenience foods likewise can contribute nutritionally to one's diet. However, why not use fresh fruits and vegetables—seasons permitting—and be sure of obtaining key nutritional factors in a more natural state. And, since you should not overcook, it will not take any more time than preparing a frozen food.

A Cure for Osteomyelitis through Proper Diet

Another early experience with nutritional therapy occurred when I received a visit from the secretary-treasurer of the country's second largest cookie and biscuit company. This gentleman had been suffering with a chronic osteomyelitis condition which is an inflammation of the bone. Other than this problem, he was in good health. He told me that the condition, which in this case was affecting his leg, had been bothering him for 18 years. At the time that I saw him, he was 40 years old. I was surprised to have him consult me and explained that I was a general practitioner and not a bone specialist. He said, however, that he would like me to tell him what I would do if the infected leg were mine. I learned that he had consulted with many physicians in Chicago and at leading clinics elsewhere. The only treatment that provided any relief was lancing the leg in order to relieve the pressure of the pus pocket. This was in 1929 when there were no antibiotics to treat such an infection.

I told him that my approach would be to treat the infection from within. This meant, I explained, altering his eating habits. The eating plan that I proposed to him is the same basic regime—with obvious adjustments to meet certain medical objectives—that I recommend to most of my patients to this day, and includes the following:

1. Protein in some form (eggs, milk, cheese, fish, meat, poultry, etc.). *Three servings daily.* It's important to select and eat from a variety of protein sources, not just meat, for example.
2. Fresh or lightly cooked vegetables. *One serving of two vegetables twice a day.* Examples: salad and zucchini equal one serving; broccoli and carrots equal one serving.

3. Fresh fruit or fruit juice. *Three servings daily.* Examples: grapefruit for breakfast; apple or pear for lunch; melon for dinner.
4. Whole-grain breads, cereals, or other grain products. *Two to three servings daily.* Example: shredded wheat for breakfast; two slices whole wheat bread with dinner.
5. Water (preferably distilled). *Six to eight glasses daily.*

I also recommended to the osteomyelitis patient that he eat liver two to three times a week. Obviously, some 55 years ago our scientific knowledge of the value of various foods was not what it is today. In recommending liver, I was doing so on the basis that back then it was regarded as an excellent food source and high in iron. I don't mean to suggest that liver alone did the trick in this case but when we examine what it furnishes, it is indeed an excellent and nutritionally important food. As a point of interest, let's see what he was receiving when he had a three ounce serving of fried beef liver. In parentheses are the adult recommended daily allowances for the nutritional factors listed:

vitamin A	45390 I.U.	(5000 I.U.)
vitamin C	23 mg.	(60 mg.)
thiamine	0.22 mg.	(1.5 mg.)
riboflavin	3.56 mg.	(1.7 mg.)
niacin	14 mg.	(20 mg.)
calcium	9 mg.	(1000 mg.)
phosphorus	405 mg.	(1000 mg.)
iron	7.5 mg.	(18 mg.)

I also prescribed a multivitamin preparation and dicalcium phosphate. Within a year the leg was healed and the osteomyelitis never returned.

How to Create the Right Nutritional Environment for Healing

In the therapeutic regime that was prescribed above, I believe that it was a combination of nutritional factors that helped clear up the condition. The important thing that resulted was that we created the right nutritional environment for the healing process to take place. Partly cooking the vegetables preserved the mineral content of these foods, the dicalcium phosphate provided calcium and phosphorus that are important in bone formation, the fruits furnished vitamin C among other factors to bolster the immune system, the liver provided plenty of vitamin A that is essential for protein metabolism in the liver and regulates the formation of cartilage, and the vitamin preparation filled in with extra nutritional assistance. The important point here, to repeat, is to create the right nutritional environment for the body's own healing powers to function.

Nutritional Approach Averts Life-Threatening Occurrence of Eclampsia

My next experience with the tremendous impact that nutritional therapy can have occurred in the prenatal clinic at Cook County Hospital. A condition that can affect pregnant women and is characterized in its most serious stage by coma and convulsions is called eclampsia. If uncontrolled it can lead to a fetal mortality rate of 20 to 25 percent and a maternal mortality of five to ten percent.

In the late 1920's and early 1930's, the cause-and-effect theory held by many physicians was that an increase in weight of the pregnant woman was related to an accompanying symptom of edema or swelling. My ideas were in the opposite direction. After observing hundreds of prenatal cases in the clinic at Cook County, it seemed to me that the edema and elevated blood pressure, which was another warning signal of the impending eclamptic crisis, was caused by an increase in weight and not the other way around. I thought that maybe it was poor diet with emphasis on fattening and high-carbohydrate, empty calorie foods that produced excessive weight gains. In turn, the blood pressure went up, edema developed and the groundwork was laid for the development of life-threatening eclampsia. With this premise in mind, I began to pay close attention to the diet of the pregnant women in the hospital and, also, in my private practice. We monitored the patients very closely to see that there was no excessive weight gain, and I was gratified to see a substantial reduction in the symptoms of high blood pressure and edema, thereby avoiding and lessening the possibility of developing the catastrophic consequences of eclampsia. I will provide a little more discussion on eclampsia in the "Female Problems" chapter.

Today, of course, obstetricians pay close attention to weight gains of their pregnant patients and establish dietary programs to avoid too large an increase. If overweight can lead to circulatory and other problems for the population at large, doesn't it follow that even more problems might arise for a pregnant woman when she puts on weight indiscriminately. The excess weight can impose a burden on her cardiovascular system at a time when it is endeavoring to provide nourishment to her body and to the developing fetus as well. The approach today, of course, is to limit weight gain to within certain limits to avoid such problems as eclampsia.

Proper Prenatal Care Produces Healthy Baby after Earlier Tragedies

The following case happened in the 1930's when I had a 30-year-old female patient referred to me. She told me about her six-year-old daughter who was constantly experiencing colds, bronchitis, and other upper-respiratory tract problems. In addition, I learned that she had given birth to two children who were afflicted with a disease that produced a wasting of skeletal muscle (then referred to as Oppenheim's Disease). One of the babies had died at three months and the other at six months of age. The patient said that she had asked a prominent pediatrician what could be done to avoid these tragic births. She was told that there was no apparent cause for this happening and that there was no remedy. With that information, the woman and her husband decided against having any more children.

In tackling the problem of her sickly daughter, I was also focusing on the mother's problem. I advised her to put her nutritional house in order for the entire family—daughter, husband, and herself. To this day I don't believe that you can stimulate one individual of a family group to eat well nutritionally and ignore the rest. If this does occur, the best motivation for the one who starts to eat well is not provided, as he sees the rest of the family indulging itself in junk or empty calorie foods. I outlined for her and her family the same basic eating plan as prescribed for the osteomyelitis patient mentioned earlier in this chapter. I urged her to prepare adequate servings of raw and lightly cooked vegetables, provide plenty of fresh fruit, and make available protein from various sources at the three principal meals of the day. Within a few months, at one of her regular office visits, she came in with her daughter and reported that the incidence of colds for her daughter had dropped significantly. She also said that she and her husband were experiencing renewed energy and feeling better generally.

It was at this time that I broached the subject of her becoming pregnant again. I explained to her that I was confident her chances of giving birth to a normal, healthy child were very good because my examination showed that she was in excellent physical condition. I also said that I had a great deal of faith in the dietary program preparing her for a successful pregnancy. I, of course, expected that she would show reluctance because of her previous tragedies. However, she did promise to discuss it with her husband and let me know on a subsequent office visit. I was naturally elated when on the next office visit she said that they would try to achieve another pregnancy. She did become pregnant and I paid very close attention to see that she remained on the dietary program and monitored her physical condition carefully. She experienced no problems during the pregnancy and I don't know if she and her husband were more happy than I was when I delivered a healthy baby girl. Later, through the years, she reported how energetic her new daughter turned out to be and that the older girl, also, was healthier and less subject to sniffles and sneezes.

What a pregnant woman eats and drinks before and during her pregnancy has a profound effect on the health of the baby. By eating and drinking the right nutritional foods and liquids, readers who are or expect to become pregnant will bestow the greatest gift you can give to any human being entering the world—good health, or at least a better than even chance for it.

I am against pregnant patients smoking or consuming alcohol, even in moderation. Drugs, of course, are out of the question. I am in complete agreement with the American Dietetic Association when they advise mothers-to-be at all stages of pregnancy to abstain from *all* alcohol—wine and beer included. They point out correctly that liquor consumption during the final months of pregnancy can be just as harmful to the fetus as during the early stages.

How My Early Experiences Shaped My Practice

The experiences recounted here focused my attention more and more during the latter years of my medical practice to the nutritional status of my patients. Orienting my patients to better and nutritionally valuable food choices as outlined in the preceding text seemed to me to complete the treatment. When patients followed my directions, it always seemed to aid the treatment of whatever problem was present. Conversely, when the patient took scant or no notice of dietary recommendations, the treatment took longer, was not as effective, or even failed more often. The medical profession, of course, recognizes this whole idea in a roundabout way when they say that this person is a good candidate for a surgical procedure and that one might not be. What they are saying, of course, is that one individual is in a good physical and nutritional state to accept the traumatic consequences of surgery. So, it should also follow that treatment less than surgical intervention ought to be more successful on people who are in good physical and nutritional condition. This has been my experience.

I have seen dramatic effects accompany simple nutritional changes. For example, it is not exaggerating to say that families can be literally torn apart by the devastating symptoms and personality changes that accompany what might be regarded as a simple problem—premenstrual tension. Severe headaches, anxiety attacks, nausea, swelling, tender breasts, crying, hysteria, and overall nervousness can crush the victim and make life difficult for those in proximity. Sedation has been a conventional type of treatment and one that takes no notice of possible nutritional deficiencies that might result from the individual's dietary regime. I have used a simple nutritional approach that has alleviated these symptoms in hundreds of my patients and this is cited in the "Female Problems" chapter. I might add that scores of husbands have expressed their thanks to me for the relief that I have afforded their wives and for the tranquility that ensued.

In the pages that follow, and the recounting of the medical problems with which I have had some success, I believe that you will come to see that when you take just a little extra effort to provide the correct nutritional environment for your body, your body will respond positively and function in the manner that will make you a happier, healthier person.

Chapter 2

Vitamin Therapy for Relieving Troublesome Health Problems and Conditions

Vitamins are organic compounds that are necessary to carry out specific and vital functions in the cells and tissues of the body. Because they cannot be made by the body, their absence or insufficient supply can result in specific deficiency conditions or diseases. The best way to obtain what the body needs in the way of vitamins is to eat from key food groups—whole cereals and grains, meats, vegetables, fruit, and dairy products. Coffee and toast in the morning, fries and a cola in the afternoon, and a TV dinner in the evening are not the way to go about it. You need something from all of the food groups mentioned.

The recommended daily allowance (RDA) differs considerably from the therapeutic dose for a vitamin. The RDA for vitamin C is given as 60 mg. or 0.06 grams daily. The therapeutic dose can range from two to three grams and upward. I take about three grams of vitamin C a day as a prophylactic dose against colds and to keep my immune system functioning as optimally as possible.

In the following discussion on vitamins, we will report what are currently considered the dietary requirements. It is important to remember that the actual amounts that, individually, we might need can vary according to age, occupation, stress under which we perform, and our individual biological makeup. If our hearts, lungs, brains, pancreas, skeletal system, and musculature were all stamped out by a machine according to the same specifications, then we might require the same amount of vitamins. If we all grew old and reacted to stress in the same manner, then the amounts given as the RDA could be accepted as the final answer to our needs. Since this is obviously not the case, we need to keep an inquiring mind as to what each of us requires in the way of vitamins, and also minerals for that matter. The discovery and research process into the role and requirements of vitamins continues. All of us interested in keeping our bodies functioning at optimum levels need to stay aware of what is occurring. Read, attend seminars, seek out nutrition-oriented physicians, eat from all food groups, and regard the RDA as a guide that is subject to change as new information comes to light.

Fat-Soluble Vitamins

The fat-soluble vitamins are A, D, E, and K. In order to be absorbed by the body and carry out their respective functions, they require some form of fat to work. In other words, don't take a vitamin A, D, E, or K capsule and wash it down with water or juice. Instead, they should be taken with a meal containing some sort of fat—buttered toast, cheese, oil, etc.

Vitamin A

Vitamin A promotes growth and repair of body tissues. In addition, new research has given it importance in the fight against cancer. Again, it is important to emphasize that the therapeutic use of vitamins should be performed only under the guidance of nutritionally competent and expert medical practitioners. Otherwise, the hoped-for results may not be attained and the real therapeutic value of vitamins will be lost.

In general, vitamin A is the most important vitamin for eye and skin health. Maintaining clear eyes and normal vision is dependent on an adequate intake of vitamin A. Therapeutic doses, of course, may vary upward from the RDA or recommended daily allowance. Vitamin A is important to the formation of visual purple which is a substance in the eye necessary for proper vision, particularly night vision. A major nutritional cause of blindness in children is attributed to extreme vitamin A deficiency.

Maintaining soft, smooth, disease-free skin is dependent on the proper nutritional intake of vitamin A. It protects specialized epithelial tissues such as the mucous membranes of the mouth, nose, and lungs. In this function vitamin A reduces the chance for infection through these vital tissues. In the absence of vitamin A, normal secretory epithelium is replaced by a dry, keratinized epithelium which is more susceptible to invasion by infectious organisms. Xerophthalmia (keratinization of ocular tissue), which may progress to blindness, is a late result of vitamin A deficiency.

"Nightblindness," impaired vision in dim light, is the classic symptom of a deficiency of vitamin A. Moderate deficiency may cause the development of dry, rough skin, dry eyelids and reddened eyes, and discomfort in bright sun without dark glasses. In extreme cases of vitamin A deficiency, there may be retarded growth, respiratory weakness, and defective formation of teeth.

Protection Against Colds. Vitamin A helps the body fight infections by strengthening the walls of cells so that viruses are not able to enter. In my practice I have found vitamin A a valuable therapeutic tool in helping my patients fight colds and sinus conditions.

Vitamin A and the Deleterious Effects of Stress. Stress is a two-edged sword. Under conditions of stress, mental or physical, we are able to function and perform beyond normal levels of activity. Many readers, undoubtedly, have stayed with a work task under emergency conditions to the point of mental or physical exhaustion. Students will cram and study before important examinations into the wee hours of the morning. We have heard or read about a person lifting or pushing aside a tremendous weight or obstacle to free a trapped person. The weight would be unmovable under normal circumstances. However, under stress, the glandular system of the body enables people to do the impossible. Unfortunately, the body subsequently needs and demands repayment in the form of additional rest, recuperation, repair, and nutrition. If this recuperative process is not allowed to occur, the body in the post-stress state is particularly vulnerable to disease and infection. Vitamin A is especially needed at this time to protect against infection. In particular, vitamin A has a beneficial effect on the thymus gland that has been shown by famed stress researcher Dr. Hans Selye to shrink under stress. The importance of the thymus is that it produces antibodies that are vital to warding off infection and disease.

Aiding Proper Liver Function. The liver is the largest organ in the body. In its healthy state, it neutralizes hormones no longer needed, synthesizes many amino acids used in building tissue, manufactures bile, detoxifies many drugs and toxins, and reduces protein into sugar and fat when required as reserve energy sources. Vitamin A plays a role in the protein-processing function that occurs in the liver. If we eat a high protein diet, it is necessary that vitamin A be taken in adequate amounts to insure that the protein is processed in normal fashion in the liver. A high protein diet can produce a vitamin A deficiency because the liver will use up whatever vitamin A is available to meet its own needs in breaking down protein and synthesizing amino acids.

Hearing Loss. Researchers have reported that because vitamin A is so important to the integrity of the walls of body cells, a deficiency of the vitamin can be responsible for hearing loss or otosclerosis. As cell walls of the tissues that make up the auditory system become tough and brittle, sound transmission is adversely affected. Here, too, vitamin A helps maintain a smooth tissue surface that improves sound transmission.

Taste Loss. People experiencing a loss of taste have recovered this sense through vitamin A therapy. We can conjecture that the vitamin has restored the integrity of the cells that make up taste buds.

Healthy Teeth and Gums. In another important role, vitamin A assists the performance of ameloblast cells that help build sound tooth enamel. Parallel to this function, vitamin A contributes to the ability of the mucous membranes to fight gum infection, thereby contributing to the sound health of the entire buccal or mouth cavity.

Sex and Vitamin A. When used in conjunction with vitamin E, vitamin A has helped restore sperm count to normal levels in the male. As a sidelight to this, male diabetics have a tendency to impotence which is greater than that of nondiabetic males. It is believed that this is due to the inability of diabetics to convert carotene to vitamin A that results in a lowering of male hormone production.

Vitamin A and Cancer. Vitamin A, or its precursor, beta carotene, has apparent anticarcinogenic properties. In this context, it should be pointed out that vitamin C along with the mineral selenium have demonstrated similar properties. Therefore, vitamin A should not be prescribed in isolation of other important nutritional factors. Rather, the rational individual will be one who assures that these vital nutrients are included in the diet along with the entire panoply of vitamins and minerals.

Sources of vitamin A are liver, fish liver oils, kidney, butter, egg yolk, milk, cheese, dark green and yellow vegetables (collard, turnip greens, carrots, squash), and fruits (peaches, canteloupe, and apricots). The recommended daily allowance is established as 5000 I.U. (international units).

Vitamin D

Vitamin D is active in every body function involving calcium and phosphorus and is also related to potassium metabolism. It is an important nutrient for infants and children because it is essential to the development of straight bones and strong teeth. In general, vitamin D promotes normal growth. It also protects the thyroid gland, helps the body to absorb magnesium and aids in the clotting of blood. Vitamin D and vitamin A together influence the body's use of cholesterol and thereby may reduce conditions that could predispose to heart disease.

Vitamin D and Colorectal Cancer. Eating foods high in vitamin D and calcium appears to reduce the risk of colorectal cancer, the second most common cause of cancer death in this country. In a study of nearly 2000 men, scientists found that those who frequently consumed foods rich in vitamin D and calcium had a rate of colorectal cancer just over one-third that of those who rarely consumed such foods. This finding was reported in the medical journal, *Lancet* (February 9, 1985).

Teen-Age Girls and Vitamin D. Vitamin D increases calcium absorption, retention, and utilization. Because of the demands of growth, vitamin D and calcium requirements are both high throughout adolescence. Teen-age girls given 1250 mg. of calcium daily and 650 units of vitamin D excreted far more calcium than they retained. When vitamin D was temporarily increased to 3900 units daily, ten times more calcium was retained. However, it should be pointed out that if this quantity of synthetic vitamin D were maintained it could be toxic.

Osteoporosis. Prolonged deficiency of calcium and vitamin D cause the skeleton to become demineralized. Many studies have shown that persons with this disease have had calcium intakes far below the recommended daily allowances. In addition, vitamin D is often totally lacking. Vitamin D, thus, is vitally important in the calcium absorption process and in preventing the ravages of osteoporosis.

Osteomalacia. This is a disease characterized by a gradual softening and bending of the bones with more or less severe pain. It is more common in women than men and often begins during pregnancy. It results primarily from a severe vitamin D deficiency. Individuals suffering from the disease recover when bile flow is stimulated by using a high protein diet and the diet includes oils, lecithin, calcium, and vitamin D.

Hypercalcemia. Although vitamin D guards the body's store of calcium from excretion and helps in its assimilation, large amounts of vitamin D in the system may result in hypercalcemia. This is a condition characterized by excessive amounts of calcium in the blood and soft tissues. Excess calcium deposits in the ends of long bones may result from an excessive amount of vitamin D. Reducing vitamin D intake to normal relieves the condition.

Rickets. Rickets is a deficiency disease that results from a lack of either vitamin D and calcium, or both, and occurs mainly in children. It is characterized by a softening of developing bones. The bones may then become bent and malformed, due to poor calcification. Prevention and reversal is accomplished by assuring the developing child of adequate amounts of calcium and vitamin D. It is also important for the pregnant mother to obtain nutrition from the proper food groups and to take vitamin-mineral supplementation as recommended by the attending obstetrician.

Heart Functioning. Calcium is vital in the proper contraction of the heart muscle and, also, skeletal muscle. Since vitamin D is crucial to the assimilation of calcium by the body, it affects heart performance due to its influence on the presence of calcium.

Bone Healing. To insure that broken bones heal with the proper deposition of calcium, it is important that vitamin D be an integral part of the diet.

Vitamin D can be obtained from foods or by exposure to sunlight. The best source is fish liver oil. Milk is generally fortified with 400 I.U. This amount meets the daily requirement for the vitamin. Egg yolk, organ meats, bone meal, tuna, salmon, and shrimp are other sources.

Vitamin E

Vitamin E, alpha tocopherol, is a fat-soluble vitamin and needs some form of fat to aid its absorption by the body. It should be pointed out that there is probably as much debate concerning vitamin E's nutritional role and benefits in humans as with vitamin C. I will summarize some of this information about vitamin E and in a following chapter present a larger discussion along with my own experiences.

One of the most important properties of vitamin E is its antioxidant action. In this function Vitamin E protects unsaturated fatty acids, vitamin C, and the other fat-soluble vitamins from oxidation with resulting loss of their nutritional benefits. One particular long-range benefit is believed by some to be the prevention and delay of the aging process of cells and bodily tissues.

Therapeutic applications reported include cardiovascular disease, certain anemias, wounds and burns, stress, sterility, varicose veins, and peptic ulcers. Vitamin E has also been reported to aid the performance of athletes.

Vitamin K

The body has a remarkable mechanism for stopping the escape of blood when we have cuts or scrapes. The process, of course, is blood coagulation or clotting. What basically happens is that a kind of fine mesh or network is manufactured that binds the red blood cells into fibrin or a clot. Circulating in the blood is a substance, fibrinogen, which is converted in a sequence of steps into fibrin. Using the biochemical terms involved, the process in simplified form includes these steps:

$$\begin{array}{l} \text{prothrombin} \longrightarrow \text{thrombin} \\ \qquad\qquad\qquad\quad \downarrow \\ \text{fibrinogen} \longrightarrow \text{fibrin (clot)} \end{array}$$

A key substance that is necessary to move the process along is vitamin K. It comes into play in the manufacture of prothrombin in the liver. A deficiency of vitamin K leads to the slowing of the rate of blood clotting. Putting it another way, if there is not a sufficient supply of vitamin K, there is a lower level of prothrombin in the blood. In operations, for example, if the surgeon has information to suspect possible bleeding problems, he can order a test measuring prothrombin. Supplementation with vitamin K can be ordered to assist in restoring normal prothrombin levels.

Vitamin K (actually vitamins K, as there are more than one) is a fat-soluble vitamin, like A, D, and E, and requires bile in order to be absorbed. Some form of fat in the diet stimulates the production of bile and, hence, the absorption of all the fat-soluble vitamins.

Heparin and dicumarol are anticoagulants, or blood thinners if you will, and are used in preventing thromboembolisms, or life-endangering blood clots. They act as antagonists to vitamin K, since their action is to reduce the amount of available prothrombin. Salicylates, as in aspirin, are also antagonists to vitamin K. As a result, when any of these substances are administered or used over a long period of time, supplementation with vitamin K may be required to allow the liver to restore prothrombin to normal levels.

Vitamin K is not to be taken on a regular, "pro-health," basis as other vitamins might be. In addition, no standard requirement has been established for vitamin K.

Excellent natural sources of vitamin K include asparagus, broccoli, cabbage, kale, spinach, turnip greens, and watercress. Other sources include beef liver, cheese, egg yolk, and green tea.

Water-Soluble Vitamins

The B Vitamins

All of the B vitamins are water-soluble and any natural excess is excreted. They are all active in providing the body with energy; they convert carbohydrates to glucose. The B vitamins are essential for maintaining the normal muscle tone of the intestinal tract and the digestion of carbohydrates. The need for the B vitamins increases during infection or stress of any kind. The B vitamins are necessary to the development and maintenance of healthy skin and hair. The vitamin B complex is perhaps the single most important factor in the health of nerves.

A critical factor about the B vitamins is that they should all be taken as a unit. They are interrelated in function, and large doses of any single B vitamin may be therapeutically useless or may result in a deficiency in the other B vitamins. The vitamin B complex cannot function satisfactorily in the absence of adequate amounts of protein. Equally important is that vitamin A is retained by the body in the presence of the vitamin B complex.

General symptoms of vitamin B deficiency are dry, rough, cracked, scaly skin, and dry, coarse hair. In addition, other symptoms of a B deficiency include fatigue, nervousness, insomnia, dizziness, headache, depression, irritability, constipation, and digestive disturbances.

Thiamine/Vitamin B-1

Thiamine or vitamin B-1 is sometimes called the "appetite vitamin" because individuals experiencing a deficiency of the vitamin report a diminished, or complete, loss of appetite. Thiamine aids in food digestion and assimilation. It is also required for changing the carbohydrates that we ingest into glucose that is used by the body to produce cellular or muscular energy.

An inadequate intake of thiamine produces incomplete carbohydrate digestion and metabolism. In addition, there results an accumulation of pyruvic acid in the blood that is a byproduct of fat metabolism. Normally, pyruvic acid combines with thiamine to produce a coenzyme necessary for the breakdown of carbohydrates. In the absence of thiamine, the concentration of pyruvic acid increases in the blood and can lead to a lack of an oxygen supply for body cells. An impairment of brain performance can result, as well as diminished concentration and learning ability. Thiamine is thus important in the oxidation process taking place in cells and promotes the optimum functioning of the nervous system, heart, and muscles.

Diabetic Coma Effects Are Reduced. Brain damage occurring during diabetic coma is less likely to occur when thiamine is part of the diet. And, of course, it is important that thiamine supplementation be in conjunction with the complete vitamin B complex.

Stress Conditions and Thiamine. Pregnancy, surgery, fever, and other stress conditions produce a need for more thiamine. In addition, more thiamine is needed when antibiotics are being taken over a long period of time and in cases of severe diarrhea. Each of these conditions affects normal metabolic processes and, as mentioned, thiamine is vital to food digestion and assimilation. Proper nourishment needs to be reinforced under conditions of stress and thiamine intake needs to be monitored and increased under the guidance of a trained nutritional specialist.

Benefits of Thiamine in Alcoholism. Probably the people most adversely affected by a thiamine deficiency are those consuming large quantities of alcohol. The consumption of alcohol affects liver functioning that, in turn, leads to reduced conversion of thiamine into thiamine phosphate, which is a key part of the chemical oxidation process. A deprivation of oxygen leads to an impairment of brain and muscular activity. Thiamine has been shown to be of value in treating alcohol neuritis, which is characterized by nerve inflammation leading to neuralgia, anesthesia, paralysis, and muscular atrophy in the region supplied by the affected nerve or loss of reflexes.

The memory loss and eventual brain destruction caused by excessive alcohol consumption may be preventable with large doses of vitamin B-1.

Evidence indicates that alcoholic psychosis, the second most common problem of alcoholics next to cirrhosis of the liver, may be caused by a genetic defect, according to Dr. Charles Scriver, professor of biology, pediatrics, and genetics at McGill University, Montreal.

It appears that vitamin B-1 may prevent the destruction of brain cells in these drinkers, Dr. Scriver reported to a genetics meeting. Because brain damage in alcoholics is so widespread and costly, some scientists have suggested adding vitamin B-1 to all alcoholic beverages to prevent cellular destruction, in an effort that would be comparable to adding iodine to salt to prevent goiters.

Individuals most vulnerable to alcoholic psychosis are whites whose ancestors came from the middle European nations. Blacks are not as susceptible to this form of psychosis because they do not have the genetic defect.

While the normal recommended allowance for vitamin B-1 is 1.5 mg. per day, drinkers with the genetic defect may have to consume 50 to 100 mg. daily to be protected from brain damage. There is no evidence that large doses of vitamin B-1 may have harmful side effects; of course, such side effects that might appear have to be weighed against the debilitating effects of the psychotic condition which is sure to develop in the alcoholic with the genetic defect.

Alcoholic psychosis is also known as the Wernicke-Korsakoff Syndrome. It is marked by short-term memory loss that forces people to fabricate stories to make up for their forgetfulness. The individual loses muscle coordination and in the advanced stages becomes totally incapacitated.

Researchers have linked the psychosis to a defect in the body's ability to make adequate amounts of an enzyme called transketolase. The enzyme is important for the metabolism of alcohol in the brain. If the alcohol is not metabolized properly, it causes damage to brain cells. Large doses of vitamin B-1 stimulate the activity of the low levels of transketolase so that it can break down alcohol. The biochemical defect appears to be dangerous only when the individual drinks alcohol.

Sea and Air Sickness. Sea and air sickness can be averted by the use of thiamine in combination with vitamin B-6, pyridoxine.

Improving Mental Ability. Some evidence indicates that supplementation of the diets of children with thiamine can improve learning ability. In one such test, a group of children receiving thiamine outperformed a control group that received no thiamine.

The requirements for adults has been established as 1.5 mg. daily. During pregnancy the need for thiamine is increased to 1.7 mg.

While it is present in many foods, thiamine is not available in any great amounts. Enrichment of bread, cereals, and rice has aided in increasing the thiamine value of these foods, along with other necessary factors such as riboflavin, niacin, and iron. Dry yeast and wheat germ are the best single sources, along with brown rice, pork, and blackstrap molasses. Other sources having small amounts of thiamine include lean meats, poultry, eggs, nuts, and fish. By themselves they are not outstanding but simply contribute as a group to meeting the requirements. The same holds true of milk, milk products, fruit, and vegetables.

Riboflavin/Vitamin B-2

Riboflavin promotes healthy skin and mucous membranes of the mouth. It is active in carbohydrate metabolism and is important in the maintenance of good vision and clear, healthy eyes. Riboflavin is necessary in the respiration of cells because it combines with enzymes to help the cells use oxygen.

Riboflavin functions as part of a group of enzymes called flavoproteins. These are involved in the metabolism of proteins, carbohydrates, and fats.

A deficiency of riboflavin results in a cracking of the corners of the mouth. Other symptoms include eye conditions, such as itching, sensitivity to light, tearing, and the appearance of broken blood vessels in the cornea.

A riboflavin deficiency in man is likely to occur in accompaniment with a lack of other members of the B-complex vitamins.

Riboflavin and Migraine. There is a suggestion that riboflavin may be effective in preventing migraine headaches.

The Better to See You With. Eye symptoms occurring when vitamin B-2 is undersupplied vary as the deficiency changes from mild to severe. Sensitivity to bright light, faulty vision in dim illumination, and eyes that water readily are noticeable first. When strained, the eyes may become bloodshot and painful on exposure to glare. If the deficiency becomes acute, the skin at the outer corners of the eyes may split while the eyes burn and become fiery red. Experimental cataracts have even been produced in animals by diets low in riboflavin.

When as little as five mg. of vitamin B-2 have been given daily, a variety of eye symptoms have been alleviated—watering, burning, and itching eyes; light sensitivity; large, dilated pupils; blurred vision; twilight blindness; inability to focus sharply; and eyestrain associated with performing close, detailed work.

Anyone attempting to apply riboflavin supplementation to eye problems should do so only in a diet that considers all vitamins and minerals.

Currently, the dietary requirements are established as 1.7 mg. for adults.

Beef or calf's liver is an outstanding source of riboflavin. Milk and milk products are also good sources. Other foods supply lesser amounts and consuming a variety of foods usually assures that the minimum requirements are met. Leafy vegetables, enriched bread and cereals, eggs, and fish furnish small amounts individually but, as a group, assist in meeting the individual's daily requirements.

Pyridoxine/Vitamin B-6

Pyridoxine is important for the breakdown and synthesis of proteins and must be present for the proper digestion and use of unsaturated fatty acids. It is needed for the production of antibodies and maintains the sodium-potassium balance that regulates body fluids. It helps the body manufacture red blood cells and promotes the normal functioning of the nervous system.

The need for vitamin B-6 increases during pregnancy and it has been used effectively to alleviate such symptoms as anemia, headaches, nausea, leg cramps, nervousness, water retention, and hemorrhoids. Adults who were given a B-6 antagonist developed dermatitis, nausea, depression, and inflammation of nerve endings. It has also been used following radiation treatment with good results. One very important use is in treating those anemias which do not respond to the use of iron alone.

Antihistamine Action. When proteins remain undigested, the amino acid histidine can be changed by intestinal bacteria into a toxic substance, histamine. This substance is found in abnormally large amounts in the blood of many allergic persons. Pyridoxine, along with vitamin C and pantothenic acid, has an antihistamine action. A deficiency of pyridoxine allows certain blood cells called eosinophils to increase abnormally, which is a characteristic feature of allergies. The therapy involved in solving food-allergy problems consists of supplementing the diet with pyridoxine, as well as vitamin C and pantothenic acid, thereby improving the digestive process and destroying undesirable intestinal bacteria.

Help for Epilepsy. Convulsions apparently identical to epilepsy have been produced in many species of animals, and in infants and adults by a pyridoxine deficiency. Pyridoxine in combination with magnesium has often proved effective in ameliorating, but not necessarily curing, the convulsive attacks. Both nutrients should be adequately supplied in the diet of every individual, particularly one who suffers from convulsions. Such symptoms as extreme sensitivity to noise, irritability, twitching, muscle spasms, apprehension, and tremors usually become apparent long before convulsions occur. If both pyridoxine and magnesium are increased as soon as any of these signs become noticeable, epilepsy could be substantially helped.

The Heart Victim. Research indicates that pyridoxine deficiency characterizes the cellular environment of people suffering from extreme atherosclerosis. As we all know, atherosclerosis is characterized by the deposition of cholesterol and other lipids in the connective tissue of the walls of the arteries. It is suggested that in many cases individuals can overcome the atherosclerotic effects of heavy fat consumption by getting more vitamin B-6 into their diets. Other evidence associating pyridoxine deficiency with atherosclerosis is the fact that the vitamin is a necessary adjunct for the manufacture of certain desirable unsaturated fatty acids.

Vaginal Inflammation. One of the most common causes of a vaginal discharge, usually accompanied by inflammation and itching, is a parasitic infection of the vagina known as trichomoniasis. Vitamin B-6 has been prescribed for severe vaginal inflammation and a number of women have reported experiencing relief, especially after applying a salve containing the vitamin.

Anemia. An anemia in which both the number of red cells and the amount of hemoglobin are decreased has been produced in infants and adults on diets deficient in pyridoxine. This anemia cannot be corrected by iron. It is ameliorated, however, by prescribing vitamin B-6, pyridoxine.

Sources of pyridoxine are brewer's yeast, liver, heart, kidney, wheat germ, and wheat bran; also bananas, prunes, raisins, peanuts, peanut butter, walnuts, and dry legumes. The recommended dietary allowance for adults is 2 mg. daily. During pregnancy and lactation, the daily recommended dosage is 2.5 mg.

Niacin

Niacin, another member of the vitamin B complex, is also a water-soluble vitamin. None of the digestive systems that take an active role in the digestion of carbohydrates can function without niacin. Niacin is effective in improving circulation and reducing cholesterol levels in the blood. It is also vital to the proper activity of the nervous system and the formation and maintenance of healthy skin. Niacin in some individuals can produce flushing, burning, and itching of the skin. As a result, niacinamide is used more often.

The Anti-Pellagra Factor. In 1725, the Spanish physician Casal described a disease, *mal de la rosa*, which was prevalent among peasants. Later in the 18th century, the Italian physician Frapoli named the disease "pellagra," which is derived from the Italian *pelle agra*, meaning "rough skin."

Pellagra is a very serious deficiency disease characterized by dermatitis, diarrhea, mental disturbances, inflammation of the mucous membrane of the mouth, and inflammation of the tongue. These symptoms are relieved, often spectacularly, by niacinamide therapy. It is important to bear in mind that vitamin deficiencies seldom occur singly, as can be illustrated by pellagra patients. Very often the patients exhibit symptoms caused by a lack of vitamins other than niacin, particularly a polyneuritis which means an inflammation of many nerves. Such a condition is treatable by thiamine administration.

Mental Health. From the preceding, it can be concluded that if niacin is helpful in treating a whole range of symptoms of pellagra, it can also be useful in ameliorating the single symptom. In the case of mental disturbances, for example, clinical researchers have shown that niacinamide therapy has indeed proved helpful. The vitamin is vital for the metabolism of brain cells and unless the nervous mechanisms have been damaged beyond repair due to the deficiency, their function returns quite satisfactorily when niacinamide therapy is used.

Alcoholism. Niacinamide therapy has proved helpful in treating alcoholism problems. A predisposition to alcoholism has been laid at the door of those individuals who have an anxiety neurosis. If the anxiety neurosis can be relieved, then, of course, we have a means of heading off the problems of alcoholism. Coincidentally, we have the tools at hand in the form of niacinamide therapy to treat the alcoholic's immediate problems.

The recommended daily allowance of niacin (most vitamin formulations list niacinamide) is 20 mg. for adults.

Liver, brewer's yeast, wheat germ, seafood, lean meats, enriched breads and cereals, and poultry are good sources.

Vitamin B-12/Cyanocobalamin

Vitamin B-12 can only be absorbed with the aid of an enzyme known as the intrinsic factor, normally produced by glands in the stomach.

In man, a deficiency of vitamin B-12 and folic acid results in pernicious anemia characterized by large blood-cell anemia and spinal cord degeneration. The anemia appears to come about because bone marrow cells are unable to form DNA, which results, in turn, from a faulty folic acid metabolism.

Vitamin B-12 is exceptionally potent. It has an activity 11,000 times that of a liver concentrate previously used to treat pernicious anemia.

Pernicious Anemia. Vitamin B-12 is essential in the control of pernicious anemia. The blood abnormalities characteristic of pernicious anemia can be corrected by folic acid but a simultaneous deficiency of vitamin B-12 causes this disease to be accompanied by an irreversible degeneration of the spinal cord. An individual lacking vitamin B-12 or one with untreated pernicious anemia develops a shuffling walk, loses the sense of position of his or her feet, and can become completely paralyzed. In pernicious anemia, the stomach has been so damaged that it can no longer produce the intrinsic factor that is vital for vitamin B-12 absorption. In such cases it is necessary to give vitamin B-12 by injection.

Menstrual Difficulties. Either a vitamin B-12 or a folic acid deficiency causes irregular and decreased, or cessation of, menstrual flow, but normal menstruation occurs as soon as the missing vitamin is furnished. Women who eat no meat and are therefore deficient in vitamin B-12 develop irregular menstruation which is easily corrected by supplementation with vitamin B-12 in company with other members of the B complex.

Sore Tongue. A smooth, shiny tongue usually indicates a deficiency of vitamin B-12 or folic acid and is corrected by supplying the missing vitamin or vitamins. Normal tongues are smooth but not shiny.

Vitamin B-12 is found in beef liver, kidney, heart, clams, and oysters. It is also available in muscle meats, poultry, milk, and cheese. The daily requirement of vitamin B-12 is six micrograms.

Folic Acid

Folic acid is part of the vitamin B complex. While folic acid occurs in many natural foods, it is easily destroyed by overcooking and exposure to sunlight, and a substantial loss of the vitamin occurs in foods stored at room temperature. Because of these factors, it may be more deficient in our diets than commonly thought.

Folic acid is necessary for the division of all body cells and for the production of the substances that carry the basic hereditary characteristics, RNA and DNA. No growth can occur without folic acid. It is an integral part of many enzymes in body cells and in this role is essential in the utilization of sugar and amino acids and the manufacture of antibodies to fight infection.

Folic acid deficiency in man results in anemia, inflammation of the tongue, gastrointestinal problems, fatigue, dizziness, mental depression, and shortness of breath. During pregnancy folic acid deficiency can result in hemorrhaging, miscarriage, premature birth, difficult labor, and infants already anemic at birth.

Folic Acid Deficiency Anemia. This type of anemia is characterized by the presence of giant red corpuscles in the blood and may result from an inadequate intake, defective absorption, or abnormal metabolism of folic acid. It occurs among pregnant women, individuals lacking stomach acid, infants and children following infections, and persons having a high consumption of refined foods and alcohol.

Individuals with this type of anemia will have symptoms of sore mouth and tongue and a yellowish skin color. It cannot be ameliorated with iron. However, within a few hours of adding one to five mg. of folic acid to the diet, the bone marrow starts producing new blood cells and the anemia disappears.

If the deficiency is due to an inadequate intake of foods containing folic acid, it is important that the diet be improved in all respects. Such anemia, though corrected by folic acid, will come back unless, in my opinion, vitamin C intake is adequate. Vitamin C increases iron absorption and the rate of hemoglobin production.

Sprue. Sprue, an intestinal disease, is characterized by sore mouth and tongue, anemia, severe diarrhea, and large amounts of fat in the stools. The villi that cover the walls of the small intestine become shortened, fuse together, or may be absent completely and in this way reduce the absorption of food to only a fraction of that of a healthy individual. Folic acid produces satisfactory results in combating the anemia and also in relieving the gastrointestinal symptoms.

Oral Contraceptives. Women taking oral contraceptives are subject to a deficiency of a number of important nutritional factors, including folic acid. Because of its importance in many physiological processes, including prevention of anemias, women taking oral contraceptives need to take a vitamin B complex supplement, along with a diet rich in foods containing the B vitamins. This will help restore losses of folic acid, B-6, and the other members of the B complex group.

Folic acid is found in green leafy vegetables, liver, kidney, whole grains, yeast, and legumes (cowpeas, soybeans, kidney beans, among others). The recommended dietary allowance for adults is 400 micrograms daily.

Pantothenic Acid

Pantothenic acid is a member of the vitamin B complex and is essential in the metabolism of proteins, carbohydrates, and fats. Pantothenic acid is required for normal growth and is involved in the production of the growth hormone, adrenal hormones, and acetylcholine. Acetylcholine is a chemical transmitter of nerve impulses. Pantothenic acid helps fight infection through aiding the formation of antibodies, promotes production of the amino acids necessary for growth and maintenance of tissue, and in the manufacture of hemoglobin, the coloring matter of red blood cells.

Symptoms of a deficiency include vomiting, abdominal distress, fatigue, insomnia, mental depression, numbness, and tingling of the extremities and cardiovascular disturbances. These signs were observed in an experimentally produced deficiency in human volunteers.

Nerve Disease. Pantothenic acid has been reported to be helpful in treating nerve inflammation and a psychosis marked by failure of memory and sometimes marked hallucinations.

Intestinal Problems. Individuals undergoing intestinal surgery can experience postoperative paralytic ileus. This is an obstruction of the bowel producing an accumulation of gas and accompanying distention. The administration of pantothenic acid has been reported to relieve the problem.

Allergies. The usual allergens are milk, eggs, wheat, and potatoes. It is reported that individuals have obtained relief from their allergies through pantothenic acid supplementation. It is conjecture on my part that what might be responsible is pantothenic acid's role as part of coenzyme A. This coenzyme is an important part of a number of food breakdown reactions and may thus help in ameliorating allergy problems.

Gout. Gout is a painful disease in which the individual feels, literally, as though he or she were stuck by thousands of needles in and around skeletal joints. These needles, which settle in the soft tissues around joints, are crystals of uric acid combined with sodium. Pantothenic acid is important in the production of the synovial fluids that keep joints lubricated. While not a cure for gout as such, pantothenic acid can be considered one factor in helping improve body chemistry to cope with the problem.

While found in many foods, the best sources of pantothenic acid are yeast, liver, kidney, eggs, whole grains, and wheat germ. The recommended daily allowance for adults is ten mg.

Biotin

Biotin, another member of the B complex, is important in the synthesis of fatty acids and in the breakdown of carbohydrates and protein. It occurs in a wide variety of foods and is also made by bacteria in the gastrointestinal tract. An experimental deficiency was produced in humans with resulting scaly dermatitis, depression, appetite loss, muscle pain, nausea, weariness, skin dryness, and cardiovascular abnormalities. The symptoms in this experiment were alleviated by injection of 150 to 300 micrograms of biotin daily for a period of three to five days.

This type of deficiency is brought about when diets include excessive amounts of egg whites.

Seborrheic Dermatitis. This condition in infants has responded to biotin therapy involving administration of oral or injected doses of five to ten mg. of biotin daily for several days.

Antibiotic-Caused Deficiency. Large doses of antibiotics, six grams of streptomycin daily for 10 to 20 days, have caused a deficiency of biotin manufactured in the intestinal tract. This can result in a dry, scaly eczema. The condition is helped by taking yogurt or acidophilus culture to replace the intestinal bacteria destroyed by the antibiotic.

Excellent sources include yeast, liver, sardines, whole grains, peanuts, legumes, and egg yolk. The recommended daily allowance for adults is 0.3 mg.

Inositol

Inositol is essential to fat metabolism. In combination with choline, it prevents the fatty hardening of arteries and protects the liver and kidneys.

Cholesterol Reduction. Lecithin is a powerful emulsifying agent and its presence in the blood acts to dissolve cholesterol deposits. When there is more lecithin in the blood than cholesterol, the actual amount of cholesterol can be high without the blood plasma getting milky or showing a tendency to produce fatty deposits. Lecithin, like cholesterol, is manufactured in our bodies. There are certain nutrients that are especially important in the manufacture of lecithin—methionine, choline, and inositol. There is evidence that an inadequate intake of these nutrients can lead to the deposition of cholesterol.

Mental Illness. While inositol may not be nutritionally essential for the body as a whole, it may have value in brain cell nutrition. It is present in some of the phospholipids in the brain and in experiments on animals, inositol has been found to have nutritional value. A nutritionally oriented psychiatrist, Dr. A. Hoffer, has used a combination of inositol and niacin to treat mental illness, especially in those individuals who cannot tolerate niacin or niacinamide in large amounts. It is assumed that inositol functions nutritionally.

Sources of inositol are lecithin, blackstrap molasses, citrus fruits, brewer's yeast, whole grains, and milk.

Choline

Choline is a natural part of colostrum, the fluid that is present before normal breast milk is produced in women. It is essential for newborn babies. In the body choline is synthesized by the interaction of vitamin B-12 and folic acid with the amino acid, methionine. Choline combines with fatty acids and phosphoric acid within the liver to form lecithin. And, as we have seen from the section on inositol, lecithin is vital in keeping cholesterol from forming deposits on arterial walls.

Liver and Kidney Health. Choline is essential for the health of the liver and kidneys. If too little choline is present in the diet, fat is deposited in the liver. This fatty condition of the liver may later lead to cirrhosis. Insufficient choline will also cause hemorrhaging of the kidneys.

Persons having abnormally high blood fat and cholesterol have been found to obtain almost twice as many calories daily from alcohol as normal individuals. Alcohol readily changes into saturated fat, often causing the amount of blood fat to double. It slows the blood flow, inhibits the utilization of fats, and increases the requirement for vitamin B-1, pantothenic acid, and choline.

Nerve Activity. Acetylcholine is well known as the chemical mediator of nerve activity. It is produced from choline and acetic acid. If there is a choline deficiency, nerve impulses to muscles can be impaired and muscle tone and activity adversely affected. The body under these conditions can be weakened and the consequences can be cardiac arrest and death.

The richest source of choline is egg yolk. Other sources are brewer's yeast, liver, kidney, wheat germ, soybeans, and lecithin.

Vitamin C/Ascorbic Acid

Ascorbic acid helps to build and maintain bones, blood, and other tissues. It is essential to the production of body proteins and to the proper utilization of iron and folic acid.

Many enzymes that are effective in wound healing are activated by ascorbic acid. The cholesterol level of the blood is also affected by adequate intake of ascorbic acid. In combination with bioflavonoids, vitamin C corrects capillary fragility and permeability by allowing normal formation of intercellular cement substances. Therefore, these two vitamins are very important in preventing hemorrhages. Ascorbic acid is, for this reason, important in maintaining firm, healthy gums. It also plays an important role in the nutrition of eye tissues.

Mild vitamin C deficiency is characterized by weariness, weakness, irritability, weight loss, and complaints of aches and pains. Prolonged deficiency may produce bleeding gums and gingivitis with loosening of the teeth. There may be a tendency to bruise and bleed easily in any part of the body, acquire swollen, painful joints, and develop the deficiency disease, scurvy.

The body's requirement for vitamin C is increased by stress. Such factors as anxiety, infection, injury, surgery, burns and fatigue accelerate vitamin C depletion. Hot weather, cigarette smoking, and industrial air pollution also speed up the use of vitamin C in the body. Exposure to cold weather increases urinary excretion of vitamin C. Exposure of food, citrus drinks, or supplements to air reduces the ascorbic acid content.

Colds. In "Vitamin C the Common Cold and the Flu," Dr. Linus Pauling cites one researcher's therapeutic regime for treating colds as involving 600 mg. of ascorbic acid as the initial dosage followed by an additional 600 mg. every three hours. This regime is to be started at the first signs of a cold—scratchiness of the throat, sneezing, nasal drip, and a chill. At bedtime the amount is increased to 750 mg. This schedule amounting to about 4 grams daily is to be followed for three to four days, reduced to 400 mg. every three hours for several days and then to 200 mg. every three hours. In this treatment schedule, it was reported that a cold that has apparently been headed off may return even after a week or more, if the ascorbic acid is discontinued abruptly.

Dr. Pauling writes: "It may be a long time before we know what the optimum rate of intake of this important food is.

There is no doubt that it varies somewhat from person to person...I am sure that an increased intake of ascorbic acid, ten to one hundred times the daily allowance recommended by the Food and Nutrition Board, leads to improvement in general health and to increased resistance to infectious disease, including the common cold.

"I am convinced by the evidence now available that ascorbic acid is to be preferred to the analgesics, antihistamines, and other dangerous drugs that are recommended for the treatment of the common cold by the purveyors of cold medicines."

Influenza. Again from the Pauling book, we have this statement: "I conclude...that the prophylactic intake of ascorbic acid, the dose taken regularly to preserve good health and provide protection against disease, almost certainly should be more than 250 mg. per day for most people. Other considerations lead me to suggest the range 250 mg. to 4000 mg. or even 10,000 mg. for recommended daily intake for most people...Such an intake should decrease the chance of contracting the common cold or influenza and, in case that the viral infection is contracted, should prevent a secondary bacterial infection from developing. Furthermore, it is my opinion that if ascorbic acid is used in the right way in the future we shall be able to avert epidemics and pandemics of influenza."

Gallstones. There is evidence to suggest that increased intake of vitamin C produces more bile acid which means that cholesterol remains in solution. In turn, this reduces the danger of gallstone formation.

Side Effects of Prescription Drugs. Work has been done showing that vitamin C counteracts the harmful side effects of potent prescription drugs that may be prescribed for a whole host of diseases and ailments. Corticosteroids, for example, are prescribed for arthritis sufferers and as side effects can produce edema, hyperglycemia, acne, congestive heart failure, hypertension, and other effects. Vitamin C given to patients taking corticosteroids has helped reduce the blocking of the infection-defense mechanism that steroid compounds produce.

Studies of the blood plasma and platelets of arthritis patients show that there is a reduced level of vitamin C in those patients who take aspirin on a daily basis. Platelets are vital in the blood clotting mechanism and important, therefore, in the event of external injury. Arthritis patients taking aspirin should supplement with vitamin C to insure proper platelet functioning in the event there is an injury with resultant bleeding.

Back Pain. It has been reported that vitamin C helps individuals with back problems. This effect is traced to the role of vitamin C in forming collagen, which helps maintain the elasticity of connective tissue. Because of the complex arrangement of the attachments of ligaments and other connecting structures throughout the vertebral column, it is vital that suppleness and elasticity be maintained. Vitamin C helps the connective tissue and other structures remain supple.

Surgery. The fact that ascorbic acid is required for the synthesis of collagen suggests that people undergoing surgery should receive an extra supplement of vitamin C. Many surgeons order the administration of extra vitamin C for their surgical patients.

Heart Disease. Collagen has structural and supportive functions that are indispensable to heart tissues and to blood vessels—and, as suggested in the preceding, to all bodily tissues. No heart or blood vessel or other organ could possibly perform its function without collagen. No heart or blood vessel can be maintained in healthy condition without vitamin C.

Unsaturated fatty substances have an important role in the functioning of cell membranes and other tissues. These substances are converted by oxidation to peroxides that are harmful. Vitamin C and vitamin E are natural antioxidants. An increased intake of these vitamins provides protection against cardiovascular disease. Vitamin E may be the more important of the two but vitamin C is also important. A proper supplementation with vitamins C and E may help to prevent premature aging, particularly if one's diet has an excess of polyunsaturated fats.

It has been found that increased intake of vitamin C decreases the concentration of cholesterol in the blood.

Cancer. Dr. Linus Pauling, who holds two Nobel Prizes, and has devoted a number of years to the study of the effects of vitamin C, estimates the probability of incurring cancer at a given age might be cut to one-quarter of the present rate if people were to take vitamin C daily in the range of one to ten grams.

A possible mechanism of the action of ascorbic acid against cancer is the stimulation of the natural immune mechanism. It is known that the probability of a favorable outcome for the cancer patient increases with an increase in the rate at which his body is able to manufacture lymphocytes. Studies have shown that an intake of five to ten grams of ascorbic acid daily increases greatly the rate of synthesis of lymphocytes that are then increasingly available to attack and destroy malignant cells.

The RDA for vitamin C is 60 mg. See next chapter for a listing of food sources of vitamin C and more information about this controversial vitamin.

As you read this review of how and where vitamins are important to us and what their natural sources are, I hope you come away with the idea that variety in food is important. There is no single, magic vitamin nor is there a single, magic food that is guaranteed to keep you and me 100 percent healthy. Each of us needs a full complement of vitamins—and minerals, of course—until in consultation with a nutritionally knowledgeable physician, we find that a particular medical problem or condition is amenable to special or enhanced nutritional therapy.

Up to that point, however, the safest bet is to eat from a wide selection of foods to meet vitamin requirements. By this I mean fresh fruits, fresh vegetables, whole grain foods, dairy products, and high quality protein in the form of fish, poultry, and lean beef.

Little-Known Foods That Are High in Nutrients

I see new and different kinds of fruits and vegetables appearing in the produce sections of supermarkets and this makes it even easier to find something to add variety to your eating for good health. Spend a little time and look for the unusual. Even ask the produce manager at your supermarket to include some different items. Eating for good health does not mean that you have to rely only on carrots, apples, and oranges. Here, for example, are a few unusual fruits and vegetables that you might look and ask for:

Cherimoya. About the size of a large softball, this fruit has a creamy, custard-like texture, and the combined flavor of pineapple, papaya, and banana. A 3½ ounce serving provides: 94 calories, protein (1.3 gram), carbohydrates (24 grams), fat (0.4 grams), vitamin A (10 I.U.), vitamin C (9 mg.), calcium (23 mg.), phosphorus (40 mg.), iron (0.5 mg.), thiamine (.10 mg.), riboflavin (.11 mg.), and niacin (1.3 mg.).

Feijoa. Also called the pineapple guava, this tropical fruit tastes like a guava with a slight strawberry and pineapple flavor. It's a good source of vitamins A and C, and potassium.

Japanese Pear. A crunchy fruit resembling a golden delicious apple but with the flavor of a bartlett pear. It has fair amounts of vitamins A and C, only 2 mg. of sodium, 61 calories, and is low in fat per 3½ ounce serving.

Jicama. A root vegetable shaped like a turnip, the Jicama has a sweet taste similar to a jerusalem artichoke. A 3½ ounce serving is 90 percent water and only 45 calories (ideal for weight-reducing diets); other nutrients include: protein (1.2 grams), carbohydrates (10.6 grams), fat (0.1 grams), vitamin A (trace amounts), vitamin C (21 mg.), calcium (18 mg.), phosphorus (16 mg.), iron (0.8 mg.), potassium and sodium (trace amounts), thiamine, riboflavin, and niacin (.03 mg.).

Plantain. A banana-like fruit that can be baked, stewed, mashed, or fried. A 3½ ounce serving has: 119 calories, protein (1.1 grams), carbohydrates (31.2 grams), fat (.04 grams), sodium (5 mg.), calcium (7 mg.), phosphorus (30 mg.), iron

(.7 mg.), potassium (385 mg.), thiamine (.06 mg.), riboflavin (.04 mg.), niacin (.6 mg.), and vitamin C (14 mg.). The white flesh variety has 10 I.U. of vitamin A, while the deep yellow flesh variety has 1200 I.U. of vitamin A.

Passion Fruit. Also known as the granidilla, it has a tart, raspberry-like flavor. It is a source of the following nutrients: 90 calories, protein (2.2 grams), carbohydrates (21.2 grams), fat (.7 grams), sodium (28 mg.), vitamin A (700 I.U.), vitamin C (30 mg.), calcium (13 mg.), phosphorus (64 mg.), iron (1.6 mg.), potassium (348 mg.), riboflavin (.13 mg.), and niacin (1.5 mg.).

Purple Cole. A cross between purple kale and cabbage, the vegetable has a mild, cabbage-like flavor. In the absence of definitive information and because it is related to kale, Purple Cole should be a good source of vitamins A and C and also have amounts of calcium, potassium, and iron.

Salsify. Popular during colonial times, this is a rediscovered rather than a new plant. It's a mild-tasting vegetable that looks like a homely carrot. Nutritionally, it is a source of calcium, potassium, and phosphorus.

Chapter 3

The Truth About the Wonder Vitamins C & E

My Clinical Experience with the Controversial Vitamin C

Controversy swirls around the therapeutic effectiveness of vitamin C.

Is it effective against the common cold? Against cancer? Against infection? Where else can vitamin C be used?

Studies about the use of vitamin C seem to run a cycle of confirming and refuting each other. In the midst of the claims, counterclaims, and disputes, all I can do is report *my* clinical experience with vitamin C.

Vitamin C and the Common Cold

It is no startling revelation to note that the common cold is responsible for a tremendous amount of human suffering. The common cold is really not very common or ordinary when you have its symptoms, including dry, scratchy, or sore throat, runny nose, sneezing, coughing, headache, chills, muscle aches, weakness, and fatigue. We all don't, of course, experience the symptoms to the same degree, and the many viruses that have been implicated can be unique in the symptoms they produce. What is serious, in addition to these symptoms, is that during the course of the cold, bacterial invaders that can lead to such major difficulties as middle ear infections, bronchitis, and pneumonia can attack the body.

In the event that a medical examination indicates that the more serious bacterial infections are developing, I prescribe an antibiotic.

I have had good results prescribing vitamin C to patients with common cold symptoms. In reporting this, I realize I stand to be contradicted. How are you, the reader, going to handle the continuing debate? You have but two people to check with the next time you have a cold and that is yourself and your doctor. If he agrees with you, determine what vitamin C can do in relieving your cold symptoms, in the event you haven't tried it already.

In my treatment course, depending on a host of factors including the severity of symptoms, I prescribe four to five grams of vitamin C daily for the first four to five days. It is possible that I may increase the dosage but, in any event, the vitamin C is to be taken in 500 mg. doses daily throughout the day. I recommend a full glass of water with each dose. Depending on the relief being experienced, the dosage is reduced to three grams daily for the next three days. Following further improvement of symptoms, I will recommend a reduction to two grams daily for another two to three days.

I wish to repeat that since there are many viruses out there, I may modify the therapy, including the vitamin C, according to the symptoms, physical condition of the patient, and other factors.

I need to caution that vitamin C is not a magic bullet to be used to the exclusion of other nutrients and sound eating habits. Plenty of other liquids, natural sources of vitamin C in fruits and fruit juices, whole grain foods to aid elimination, a multivitamin, and a mineral supplement are needed to help the body beat back the "common" cold.

In the patients that I have treated, vitamin C helps relieve the symptoms of a cold.

A typical case is that of an attorney friend of mine who was experiencing all of the flu symptoms, including runny nose, chest congestion, and severe coughing episodes. He told me that he was taking an antibiotic prescribed by another physician and obtaining no relief. Antibiotics are not effective against viral infections and, as mentioned, can only protect against the development of more severe problems of bacterial origin. I prescribed four grams of vitamin C daily and within 48 hours, he began to experience relief of the symptoms.

I estimate that this therapeutic approach has proved effective in 60 percent of the several hundred cases of flu on whom I have tried the therapy.

Vitamin C and Urinary Tract Infections

An interesting medical problem is that of chronic bladder infection where the patient has frequent urination and burning. Upon laboratory analysis of the urine, definite pus cells can be found in an amount pointing to an infection. One treatment that I have used that helps these patients is acidifying the urine. One of the finest acidifying agents that we have for this purpose is vitamin C. In my experience, the use of one or two 500 mg. vitamin C tablets, three times daily, usually accomplishes the objective within four or five days. I have found the time-release vitamin C capsules to be the most effective in treating the problem.

I remember being in my optometrist's office having my prescription for glasses renewed. He started to tell me about the problems he was having with bladder and urinary infections. He complained about having to be admitted to the hospital so often to have the infection treated. I prescribed four grams of vitamin C daily, in addition to recommending a multivitamin and mineral formula plus a balanced and nutritional diet. When he came to my office about two months later, he reported that the infection had cleared up and was pleased about not having to check into the hospital anymore.

Vitamin C and Mononucleosis

Mononucleosis is a viral infection for which there is no specific treatment. On the other hand, I have found that the condition can respond favorably to vitamin C therapy. In a number of cases I have seen the course of the infection considerably ameliorated with vitamin C treatment in the four to five grams per day range. One of my patients was a young high school girl, 16 years of age, who was positively diagnosed as having mononucleosis. We made sure with her mother that the girl started to follow a well-rounded and nutritious eating plan, multivitamins and minerals, and a prescription of four grams of vitamin C daily. Within a week's time her elevated temperature dropped, her strength returned and she was able to return to school. This quick recovery was unusual because mononucleosis leaves people debilitated for a long period of time.

Vitamin C and Herpes Simplex

I have had good results treating herpes conditions with vitamin C. This is especially true of herpes simplex which affects the lips and, also, the vulva. In these particular cases, I have the patients make a paste of vitamin C and apply directly to the affected part. It is truly remarkable how the vitamin C paste acts to dry the cysts and stop the infection. The idea of the vitamin C paste occurred to me a few years ago when I became convinced that vitamin C combats viral infection. A herpes simplex developed on my lip and I took some vitamin C tablets, crushed them and made a paste with water. I applied this to the cyst and very shortly the swelling subsided, dried up, and disappeared. If crushing the tablets becomes a messy proposition, then an alternative is to purchase sodium ascorbate powder. With the powder in a cup or saucer, add a little water and make up the paste. It is very convenient, easy, and effective to apply in this manner.

Vitamin C Aids Iron Absorption and Blocks Nitrosamine Formation

Research indicates other potential health benefits from vitamin C, including increased absorption of nonheme iron, blocking formation of nitrosamines, and overcoming the negative effects of iron absorption when soybean protein is substituted for meat in diets.

Research by Dr. Leif Hallberg of the University of Goteberg, Sweden, shows that when a typical meal of meat and two vegetables is cooked and then kept warm, the amount of vitamin C is reduced significantly. His studies indicate that when a meal is kept warm for four hours, vitamin C content is reduced approximately 76 percent. The tests also show that the absorption of nonheme iron by the body—believed to be related to vitamin C availability—is also reduced 42 percent.

The availability of meat substitutes in the form of soy protein has raised the question of a possible reduction in the absorption of vital iron. Research indicates that substituting soy protein for meat does indeed reduce iron absorption. However, if the meat substitute is fortified with vitamin C, which increases iron absorption, the net effect is positive; there is a higher absorption of iron.

Dietary studies with volunteers demonstrate that adding small amounts of vitamin C to a meal, 50 mg. for example, can increase the absorption of iron from three to six times. The main effect is on nonheme iron that we obtain from vegetables and cereals, as opposed to heme iron which is obtained from the hemoglobin and myoglobin in meat. Nonheme iron forms the major part of the iron intake.

In further research on how vitamin C is lost, one survey of meals in 150 British hospitals showed that no vitamin C remained in the food by the time it was served in two hospitals and that in the majority of the remaining hospitals, the level had dropped below the minimum of 30 mg. recommended in the United Kingdom.

Both vitamins C and E act as antioxidants and are effective in blocking the formation of nitrosamines which have been implicated as cancer-causing agents. Vitamin C, because it is water soluble, is stored however briefly in the lean portion of the body, while fat-soluble vitamin E is stored in the fatty portions of the body. Sodium nitrite in bacon is of particular concern because it can be converted in the intestinal tract into potentially lethal nitrosamines. While it is obviously best to eliminate bacon and similarly smoked meats from the diet, those who cannot should assure themselves adequate amounts of both vitamins C and E to cope with the formation of nitrosamines.

Vitamin C Helps Wound Healing in Surgery

Because ascorbic acid is needed for the synthesis of collagen which is the cement of connective tissue and bones, and because wounds in people suffering from scurvy fail to heal properly, it is suggested that surgical patients ought to receive extra amounts of vitamin C. Some investigators have reported that surgical wounds do not heal in patients whose blood plasma concentration of ascorbate is less than two mg. per liter. This indicate a consumption of less than 20 mg. per day.

Some observations by physicians point to a decrease in postsurgical pain and the length of hospitalization when vitamin C is given in adequate amounts.

Vitamin C Helps in Cardiovascular Disease

Unsaturated fatty substances play a key role in biochemical functioning in cell membranes and other tissues. The fatty substances are changed into harmful peroxides. Because vitamins C and E are natural antioxidants, an increased consumption provides a line of defense against heart disease. The two vitamins may also help to prevent premature aging, particularly if an individual's eating habits overemphasizes food high in polyunsaturates.

It has been found that an increased intake of ascorbic acid acts to reduce cholesterol in the blood. One researcher working with a group of subjects who had an average cholesterol level of 253 mg. per decliter found that one gram ascorbic acid per day had the effect of lowering the cholesterol level to 210 mg. per decliter after six months.

Vitamin C—Help in Pregnancy

It has been known for over 30 years that pregnant women need more vitamin C than other women. Part of the reason for this extra need is that the developing fetus requires a good supply of vitamin C and there is a mechanism in the placenta for transferring vitamin C from the blood of the mother into that of the fetus. A low value of vitamin C in the blood has been shown to be correlated with the incidence of hemorrhagic disease of the newborn.

Other research shows that an adequate intake of vitamin C is important in controlling threatened, spontaneous, and habitual abortion. In addition to vitamin C, the patient group received bioflavonoids and vitamin K, and a 91 percent success rate in avoiding the abortion problem was achieved.

Sources of Vitamin C

Food sources with better than average vitamin C content include the following. As a point of reference, the RDA for vitamin C is 60 mg.

avocado, raw, one	43 mg.
cranberry juice, one cup	81 mg.
grapefruit, raw, one-half	44 mg.
grapefruit juice, one cup	93 mg.
cantaloupe, raw, one-half	90 mg.
orange, raw, one	66 mg.
orange juice, one cup	124 mg.
strawberries, raw, one cup	88 mg.
broccoli, raw, one cup	140 mg.
brussels sprouts, raw, one cup	135 mg.
cabbage, raw, one cup	42 mg.
cauliflower, raw, one cup	90 mg.
collards, raw, one cup	144 mg.
kale, raw, one cup	102 mg.
peppers, sweet, raw, one pod	94 mg.
spinach, raw, one cup	50 mg.
tomato juice, one cup	39 mg.
turnip greens, raw, one cup	68 mg.

The Protective Power of Vitamin E and How It Can Work for You

Of eight naturally occurring compounds that have vitamin E activity, alpha tocopheral is the most active form. The most important sources of the tocopherols are the various vegetable oils. Safflower oil has one of the highest concentrations of alpha tocopherol. Throughout the remainder of this chapter in mentioning vitamin E, we will be referring to alpha tocopherol.

How Vitamin E Helps the Body

Vitamin E is essential for protecting the integrity of that structure called the cell membrane, which surrounds the contents of human body cells. Cell membranes are composed primarily of lipid, or fat, and protein molecules. Vitamin E acts as an antioxidant in protecting the lipid molecules which make up the mosaic-type configuration of the cell membrane. In this manner vitamin E is responsible for the proper functioning of all the cells of all body systems, including respiratory, circulatory, nervous, digestive, and excretory.

Vitamin E helps protect the body against pollution products and poisons that result from the breakdown of organic substances. Persons living in highly industrialized areas may very well require extra supplementation with vitamin E.

Recent findings indicate that vitamin E may play an important role in helping the body fight cancers.

Vitamin E protects polyunsaturated fatty acids (PUFA) from oxidation. An adequate intake of vitamin E is necessary if you have reoriented or are reorienting your diet to include more PUFA.

In acting as a detoxifying agent and antioxidant, vitamin E may prevent or slow the aging of cells and tissues.

Vitamin E may help the body cope with physical and mental stress.

How Adequate Is Our Vitamin E Intake?

I think it's important that we all analyze our intake of vitamin E because of what has happened to its content in foods during the past few decades. Even the best of diets may contain only five to ten International Units per day, compared to an average of 100 I.U. at the turn of the century. Large losses of alpha tocopherol occur during commercial processes. For example, in making wheat flour, alpha tocopherol is lost when the bran and sperm are separated. In addition, almost all of the remaining alpha tocopherol is lost if chlorine dioxide is used in the bleaching process to make white flour.

Even vegetable and seed oils lose alpha tocopherol in various purification and hydrogenation steps.

Vitamin E is unstable in the presence of air. Other factors that reduce its biological activity are sunlight, heat, and lead and iron salts.

Because of these factors affecting its availability, I think supplementation with at least 100 I.U. daily is a good idea. Many multivitamin and mineral formulations provide at least part of this amount.

Vitamin E's Role in the Prevention of Heart Disease

I'll begin by saying that, in my opinion, anyone over the age of 40 should take vitamin E prophylactically to form a line of defense against heart disease.

The therapeutic value of vitamin E in treating problems of the cardiovascular system is a controversial one. Some investigtors have obtained good results in treating patients and others have not. I happen to believe that vitamin E has value when prescribed for patients in the right dosage at the right time. Ideally, of course, I would rather see people reorient eating habits, so as to include adequate amounts of vitamin E and other necessary nutritional factors instead of reaching the point where vitamin E is required in therapeutic amounts. Part and parcel of the reorientation process, to be sure, is a change of lifestyle to eliminate those debit entries which include smoking, drinking, lack of rest, etc.

Vitamin E functions as an anticlotting agent and may be helpful, too, in dissolving existing clots. When it is present in normal amounts, abnormal clotting is less likely to occur. If given at the very onset of an attack of coronary occlusion, there is some evidence that it will help dissolve clots and minimize the death of cardiac muscle deprived of its blood supply. Experiments have demonstrated that vitamin E augments the action of pharmaceutical blood thinners. In contrast to these blood thinners, however, vitamin E provides the benefit of not producing bleeding tendencies.

Vitamin E also works to decrease the oxygen requirements of the heart muscle and, in this way, minimizes the extent of damage occurring from a coronary occlusion.

In another aspect of its action, vitamin E improves the ability of red blood cells to transport oxygen. Male subjects on a vitamin E-deficient diet showed an increase in hemolysis. This is a loss by red blood cells of their hemoglobin which is the oxygen-carrying portion of red blood cells. By helping to keep intact the oxygen-carrying capacity of the blood, vitamin E assists any damaged heart muscle supplied with vital oxygen.

In another of its beneficial actions, vitamin E helps open up additional or collateral circulation to damaged heart muscle.

One area of its action on the cardiovascular system where there seems to be agreement is vitamin E's role in relieving peripheral vascular disease. Patients with the problem were treated with vitamin E compared with vasodilators, anticoagulants, or a multiple vitamin preparation. Those on vitamin E were improved in the capacity to walk distances, withstand distress, or pain, and there was also a reduction in legs amputated as a result of gangrene.

Vitamin E has been used in treating angina attacks. My most important success in this regard is a physician colleague whose case I recount in the "Open an I.H.A." chapter. Here was a physician barely able to walk and whose deteriorating condition was dramatically reversed by vitamin E.

In my practice I have seen positive results from vitamin E supplementation in well over 100 patients in the 55, 60, 65-and-over age brackets. These were patients with complaints of depleted energy reserves, shortness of breath, and general tiredness. Where diagnostic tests ruled out other possibilities and pointed to diminished cardiac performance, patients placed on vitamin E responded positively and reported increased energy and ability to work longer. In a few cases where there was an elevated blood pressure, it was interesting to note that there was a return to normal readings.

Other Reported Roles for Vitamin E

Vitamin E may also protect the structure and function of muscle tissue. Various stages and forms of muscle degeneration and lesions have been found in patients with low levels of vitamin E in the blood.

It is reported that vitamin E has value in kidney disease, such as nephritis. The idea is advanced that it improves diuresis and, thus, reduces excess water in the tissues.

I think that one of its more important functions is in helping the elderly retain mental sharpness. This is related to its role in the cardiovascular system. By helping provide brain cells with oxygen-rich blood, it keeps important centers of the brain functioning. In addition, it helps ward off strokes by keeping the blood vessels open.

Treatment for Skin Scarring

Vitamin E has been cited as a treatment for skin scarring resulting from any number of causes—burns, cuts, abrasions, etc. I have had satisfactory results using vitamin E suppositories in treating the scarring of vaginal mucosa resulting from radium treatment of cancer. I had the idea that using vitamin E vaginally would soften the mucosa which was scarred and retracted by the heavy use of radium in treating cervical cancer.

One of my first cases was that of a 50-year-old female who had not been previously married. She had received a course of treatment of both radium and cobalt for cervical cancer. On examination it was found that the vaginal mucosa had retracted as a result of treating, causing vaginal dryness. The patient was about to be married and it was realized that, under the circumstances, marital relations would be painful and difficult. I prescribed vitamin E suppositories. After three to four weeks of their use an examination disclosed that the vaginal mucosa softened considerably. It was gratifying to see that the patient was now in an improved state of mind and not harboring any fears about sexual problems that might occur in her impending marriage. In a follow-up visit to the office after her marriage, she advised that she was able to have marital relations without pain or discomfort.

Another patient, 45 years of age, had also undergone treatment with radium and cobalt for cervical cancer. Examination showed that not only was the vaginal mucosa scarred but that bleeding would occur upon manipulation. I prescribed vitamin E vaginal suppositories and in the span of six weeks, the scarring became less pronounced. Further, it was noted that there was no bleeding on examination.

Vitamin E's Role in Treating Effects of Diabetes

Vitamin E proves helpful in treating the effects of diabetes mellitus that, as is commonly known, results when the body is unable to properly metabolize carbohydrates due to insufficient insulin production. Those whose lives have been saved by insulin treatment face the risk of the complications arising from the narrowing of blood vessels with consequent reduction in oxygen supply to tissues and organs. Premature arteriosclerosis, strokes, kidney disease, cataracts, peripheral artery disease, blindness, and high blood pressure are some of the hazards that diabetics face. These complications are related to how long a person has had the disease and how well it is being controlled. By its action in helping the cardiovascular system function optimally, vitamin E can be a valuable adjunct to the complete treatment of diabetes mellitus—as important as the diet which is prescribed and the insulin that must be taken.

How Vitamins A, C, E, and Selenium Work Together

Vitamin E has a sparing action on vitamin A and carotene. For example, vitamin A and carotene are more effective in curing their deficiency symptoms, if vitamin E is given simultaneously. Because vitamin E is an antioxidant, it prevents the oxidation of other easily oxidized substances, particularly fats and vitamin A. In turn, the antioxidant properties of vitamin E are enhanced by vitamin C and selenium. I use a supplement that combines all four of these antioxidant factors.

Sources of Vitamin E

It is interesting that as one reviews textbooks on nutrition, information about food sources of vitamin E is somewhat sketchy and, even conflicting. An explanation for this is that the assay of vitamin E has been a difficult procedure. In addition, oxidation and food processing destroys the vitamin E content of foods. Thus, a food stored for a long period of time, exposed to heat, air and/or light, or subjected to various processing steps, such as the bleaching of wheat flour to make it white, will show different levels of vitamin E activity, depending on when the analysis is done. Now, newer analytical instrumentation and methods, and more testing by many research groups, have improved the reliability of information about vitamin E content of foods.

In selecting better-than-average food sources of vitamin E, the focus is on those with higher alpha tocopherol content. It shows the greatest biologic activity.

In general, and this applies to most nutritional factors, the closer to the fresh and natural state you can eat a food, the more vitamin E you will add to your diet. For example, when wheat flour is bleached, it can lose up to 65 percent of its vitamin E content. Dark rye flour has three times more vitamin E than light rye. A whole, raw apple has twice the vitamin E content than just the flesh. This is another reason why it's important to eat the skin. The foods marked with an * are particularly high in vitamin E.

Vegetables

asparagus, raw*
cabbage, raw
dandelion leaf, raw
mustard greens, raw
parsley, raw
potato, sweet, raw*
turnip greens, raw*

Fruits

avocado, raw
blackberry, raw*
mango, raw

Cereal Grains

corn
oats
rice
rye
whole wheat
wheat germ*

Eggs

yolk

Vegetable/Seed Oils

cottonseed
palm
safflower
sunflower*
wheat germ oil*

Nuts/Seeds

almond*
brazil nut
filbert*
peanuts
pecan
sunflower seed*

As far as obtaining vitamin E, alpha tocopherol, from natural or synthetic sources, there is some evidence to suggest that natural alpha tocopherol has increased activity over the synthetic form. In looking at vitamin E supplements, the natural vitamin E has a single letter *d* preceding alpha tocopherol. Synthetic vitamin E has both the letters *dl* as a prefix, for example, *dl*-alpha tocopherol.

Chapter 4

Beyond Vitamins— The Golden Nutrients You Must Have for Increased Health and Vitality

What You Can Learn from Studying Your Body's Responses

Nutrition is still quite young as a science. Research is continuing to unlock the secrets of how the body utilizes not only vitamins, but also minerals, enzymes, amino acids, and other nutritional factors. For example, a report from a meeting of the American College of Surgeons tells of the discovery that one of the amino acids, arginine, stimulates the immune response system of healthy people. The direction of further research with this amino acid is to see if it will help people with depressed immune systems fight infections and cancer.

The amazing thing about keeping up to date about nutrition is that it is not a complicated process. You don't have to buy equipment, instruments, or textbooks. You don't have to take courses. You don't have to listen to lectures. Really, all you have to do is to study your body's reaction to foods. You start by assuring yourself that you are including the basic food groups in your daily diet. Then, if an extra piece, bite, or swallow of some food or drink brings discomfort, don't immediately seek to relieve the symptom by reaching for an antacid. Often, just drinking water may produce relief because water is the universal solvent and it serves to dilute the effect of the offending food. And, just as the "wet paint" sign teaches you not to touch, learn to pay attention to and monitor the signs and signals that your body continually sends out.

The Balanced Diet

The foundation of a balanced diet includes carbohydrates, protein, fat, fiber, water, minerals, and vitamins. You might ask why I tack on minerals and vitamins when the general assumption is that foods should supply these valuable nutrients. Of course, the reason is that I don't believe that any of us can so accurately construct a diet that our daily requirements of vitamins and minerals are faithfully met. Also, special demands and stresses, medical problems and conditions, and other such factors can require vitamins and minerals above the minimum daily requirements or RDA. Therefore, as I emphasized in previous chapters, I believe in supplementation.

I do not like to use formulas as far as constructing diets is concerned. It becomes self-defeating in the long run because if people feel that they are not adhering to certain percentages or numbers, they get discouraged and revert to an indiscriminate eating plan. However, you will undoubtedly detect on my part, when I mention "well-balanced" diets, a bias in favor of protein. If I were to use a percentage formula, it might look something like this:

protein	45%
carbohydrate	35%
fat	20%

The reason for the greater bias in favor of protein is that the patients (and they are mainly female) who have come to the office have already tilted the formula heavily in favor of carbohydrates and fats. In case after case, as I have delved into the patient's eating habits, I have found a distressing pattern of a roll, donut, or toast and coffee for breakfast, perhaps a piece of pie for lunch, or no lunch at all, and finally a dinner with some protein in it. Thus, as a result of the patients that I have talked to and treated, my recommendations have tended to stress protein and reduce empty calorie carbohydrates and high-fat foods. It seems to me that with an estimated 60 million overweight people in the country, I don't think we have much of a problem as far as people consuming carbohydrates and fats is concerned. For example, a 25 gram donut has 13 grams of carbohydrate, five grams of fat, one gram of protein, and the remainder in the form of water. The problem facing us is not the complete avoidance of any kind of carbohydrate and fat, but in selecting and consuming carbohydrates with nutrient value such as whole wheat bread, dressing with a low content of saturated fat, or the many delicious fruits and vegetables available.

To put more "balance" into the diets of my patients required more of a tilt in the direction of foods with a higher protein content. This turned out to be something quite as simple as substituting a soft boiled egg, a slice of whole wheat bread, and a half glass of milk instead of the usual donut and cup of coffee for breakfast. Please remember that the calories that our bodies need can come from carbohydrates, fat, and protein. However, the protein and the important amino acids that are required need to come from protein.

The preceding thoughts and views, to repeat, are based on experiences with patients that I have seen. Whether this information applies to you depends on many factors. You should consult with a nutrition-oriented medical practitioner for an evaluation of general health, medical problems, age, occupation, level of activity, and so on. Generally speaking, however, as you do seek out foods with higher protein level, you will find that they also furnish carbohydrates and fat. Thus, it is not as though you will consume protein to the exclusion of other necessary nutrients. In the Appendix is a chart that provides a very rough caloric content of carbohydrates, fat, and protein found in a fairly small range of foods. The information has been derived from a publication of the United States Department of Agriculture, Home and Garden Bulletin Number 72, "Nutritive Value of Foods," revised April 1981. This is a very valuable bulletin to have because it provides information not only on protein, fat, and carbohydrate content of virtually all foods, but, in addition, shows values for calcium, phosphorus, iron, potassium, vitamin A, thiamine, riboflavin, niacin, and ascorbic acid (vitamin C). For example, you will find out that one cup of collard greens can furnish an amazing 14,820 I.U. of vitamin A and 144 mg. of vitamin C. The bulletin is a must for the nutritionally conscious person.

Carbohydrates—Your Fuel for Healthy Living

Carbohydrates are the major source of food energy for most people. In addition, if carbohydrates are deficient in the diet, protein is converted into fuel. When this happens, the body may not have enough protein to build tissue and muscle. In this way, carbohydrate spares protein for its more important role.

Carbohydrates are divided into two general groups: simple carbohydrates (sugars) and complex carbohydrates (starches, dextrin, cellulose, and glycogen).

Simple carbohydrates contain a single sugar unit, a monosaccharide (glucose or fructose, for example) or two sugar units, disaccharides (sucrose, maltose, or lactose).

Glucose. Glucose, also called dextrose, occurs in fruits, vegetables, and honey. It is the form of sugar to which all other carbohydrates are changed for transport in the blood and use by the tissues of the body.

Fructose. Sometimes called levulose or fruit sugar, fructose is found in honey, vegetables, and fruit, especially berries.

Sucrose. The ordinary granulated, powdered, or brown sugar which is found in sugar cane, sugar beets, molasses, and maple syrup is sucrose. It is composed of fructose and glucose.

Lactose. Lactose, or milk sugar, is formed in the mammary glands of lactating mothers, human or animal. It is a relatively expensive form of sugar, less soluble, less sweet, and more slowly digested than the other disaccharides. An undigested residue of lactose in the large intestine or colon has a laxative effect, and an excessive amount may result in diarrhea.

Maltose. Sometimes called malt sugar, this disaccharide is found in malt and malt products. It is manufactured by the action of diastase, a plant enzyme in sprouting grains, in starch. Because it is readily soluble and not readily fermented in the digestive tract, maltose is often used in combination with dextrin in infant formulas.

Starch. Starch, a complex carbohydrate, is found in grains, legumes, and vegetables. For example, potatoes are mostly starch and water.

Dextrin. When starch is digested, dextrin is the intermediate breakdown product. Digestion continues until glucose remains.

Cellulose. This sugar is the indigestible framework of plants. The indigestibility of cellulose is its main advantage to us because the undigested fiber provide the roughage or bulk in our diet for normal peristalsis (muscular contraction) of the intestines and thereby aids the elimination process.

Glycogen. Glycogen, sometimes called "animal starch," is the reserve form of carbohydrates in humans. About one-third of carbohydrates are stored as glycogen in the liver. It serves as a ready source of glucose when needed.

Complex carbohydrates are important food choices for the diet because they are usually low in fat and contain no cholesterol. In addition, carbohydrate sources such as vegetables, when not subjected to too much cooking, baking, or frying, are important sources of vitamins and minerals. Fruits are excellent sources of carbohydrates not normally subject to preparation processes that would rob them of nutritional value.

Nutritional authorities recommend that no less than 100 grams of carbohydrates are needed daily by the average adult. These carbohydrates equal approximately 400 calories and assist the body in avoiding excess protein depletion and prevent developing the condition called *ketosis.* When this occurs, it is a signal that the individual is on the verge of coma.

Despite the importance of carbohydrates, an excess in the form of sugar may result in obesity and dental problems. An effect of a diet rich in sweets, especially between meals, is the tendency to limit the consumption of other foods that are sources of necessary nutrients, vitamins, minerals, and amino acids.

If I were to make a general recommendation for normal diets, I would say a consumption of carbohydrates in the range of 225–250 grams (900–1000) calories would meet requirements of the average adult.

Selecting any carbohydrate source will rather quickly allow you to reach these levels. The summary table below shows gram and calorie values of some foods commonly found in the American diet. The intelligent course of action for all of us is to favor cereal grains, vegetables, and fruits, in order to obtain needed minerals, vitamins, and roughage, as opposed to just obtaining a full feeling from eating a bag of potato chips.

	Serving	Wt. in Grams	Carbohydrate in Grams	Calories
sugar, white	1 teaspoon	4	4	15
pizza, cheese	⅛ of 12″ pie	60	22	145
popcorn, popped, plain	1 cup	6	5	25
spaghetti, cooked	1 cup	140	32	155
pancakes	1 cake	27	6	55
bread				
white	1 slice	23	12	65
whole wheat	1 slice	25	12	60
cereal				
oatmeal	1 cup	240	23	130
shredded wheat	1 biscuit	25	20	90
cookies				
oatmeal	2 cookies	26	19	117
fruit				
apples	1 apple	212	31	125
bananas	1 banana	119	26	100
oranges	1 orange	131	16	65
vegetables				
broccoli, cooked	½ cup	78	3.5	20
carrots, 7½″ × 1⅛″	1 carrot	72	7	30
lettuce, pieces	1 cup	55	2	5
potatoes, baked	1 potato	156	33	145
potato chips	10 chips	20	10	115

The Magic of Fiber

Nonutilizable carbohydrates are such things as cellulose, lignin, gums, and agar-agar. These constitute a large part of the fiber of food, which is the indigestible part that provides bulk to the feces. The diet must contain such substances, otherwise there is a tendency for constipation to occur. Rather recently, the lack of dietary fiber has been suggested as a cause for the high incidence of colon cancer. The lack of dietary fiber is attributed to the tendency in food processing toward greater refinement with the result that the fiber is lost.

In addition, the lack of dietary fiber may be responsible for hernias of the gastrointestinal tract, hemorrhoids, gallbladder disease, appendicitis, varicose veins, and obesity. Experimental evidence suggests that fiber may bind cholesterol into a complex that aids the reduction of the cholesterol level of plasma and body tissue.

Fruits contain cellulose and are a good source of this important food factor. To be more specific:

oranges	bananas	grapes
grapefruit	pineapples	cherries
apples	prunes	blueberries
tangerines	strawberries	raspberries
pears	plums	

Bananas are an important dietary recommendation in this subject area because of the pectin content. Pectin absorbs water and provides a substantial amount of bulk plus possessing a nonirritating fiber.

Whole grain cereals and breads are important fiber sources. Under this heading are the bran cereals, shredded wheat, wheat germ, and whole wheat bread.

In the vegetable category, high-fiber sources include spinach, cabbage, carrots, celery, lettuce, asparagus, broccoli, cauliflower, and green beans.

Fat—The Crucial Difference between Saturated and Unsaturated Fatty Acids

While fats have been under attack in the dietary recommendations of many nutritionists, they do perform a number of functions. Fats slow the emptying time of the stomach because they are slower to digest. Fats serve as a reserve supply of stored body energy. Fats are an integral part of cell membranes. As we all observe, fat people seem to withstand cold better than thin people; the thicker layer of fat under their skin insulates their bodies against the cold. Conversely, however, that fat in warm weather serves to keep the body from releasing a build-up of heat. Necessarily, then, we see fat people sweating more profusely in order to maintain the optimum body-temperature level of 98.6 degrees.

Fatty tissue also forms a cushion around vital organs, such as the heart, and protects the organs against jolts, jars, and other types of physical activity that the body is subjected to.

Not only do they constitute a reserve supply of fuel or energy, fats are also efficient in the way they provide energy. For example, the same amount of fat will furnish twice the amount of energy as equivalent amounts of carbohydrates or protein.

As mentioned previously, fat serves as a transport medium for the fat-soluble vitamins, A, D, E, and K.

The following chart* compares the protein, fat, and fatty acid (saturated and unsaturated) content of servings of a few fish, beef, pork, and poultry products. Note, for example, that a three ounce serving of shrimp furnishes 21 grams of protein and 0.1 grams of saturated fat. On the other hand, a three ounce serving of sirloin steak (lean and fat) has 20 grams of protein and 11.3 grams of saturated fat. However, by trimming the fat from steaks and chops, you can approach the lower fat content of fish and chicken.

The chart also includes a comparison of margarine, butter, and vegetable oils.

I want to direct the reader's attention to linoleic acid which is one of the three most active unsaturated fatty acids (linolenic and arachidonic are the other two) and is important in the biosynthesis of prostaglandins. In turn, prostaglandins have the ability to lower blood pressure, regulate acid secretion of the stomach, regulate body temperature, and control inflammation and vascular permeability.

---

*Information is derived from Home and Garden Bulletin No. 72, "Nutritive Value of Foods," revised April 1981 and published by U.S. Dept. of Agriculture.

		Protein	Fat	Fatty Acids Saturated (Total)	Unsaturated Oleic	Unsaturated Linoleic
salmon, canned	3 oz.	17 gm.	5 gm.	0.9 gm.	0.8 gm.	0.1 gm.
shrimp, canned	3 oz.	21 gm.	1 gm.	0.1 gm.	0.1 gm.	Trace
tuna, canned	3 oz.	24 gm.	7 gm.	1.7 gm.	1.7 gm.	0.7 gm.
steak, sirloin, lean & fat	3 oz.	20 gm.	27 gm.	11.3 gm.	11.1 gm.	0.6 gm.
steak, sirloin, lean	2 oz.	18 gm.	4 gm.	1.8 gm.	1.6 gm.	0.2 gm.
pork chop, lean & fat	2.7 oz.	19 gm.	25 gm.	8.9 gm.	10.4 gm.	2.2 gm.
pork chop, lean	2 oz.	17 gm.	9 gm.	3.1 gm.	3.6 gm.	0.8 gm.
chicken, breast	2.8 oz.	26 gm.	5 gm.	1.4 gm.	1.8 gm.	1.1 gm.
margarine	1 pat	Trace	4 gm.	0.7 gm.	1.9 gm.	1.1 gm.
butter	1 pat	Trace	4 gm.	2.5 gm.	1.0 gm.	0.1 gm.
corn oil	1 tbsp.	0	14 gm.	1.7 gm.	3.3 gm.	7.8 gm.
olive oil	1 tbsp.	0	14 gm.	1.9 gm.	9.7 gm.	1.1 gm.
safflower oil	1 tbsp.	0	14 gm.	1.3 gm.	1.6 gm.	10.0 gm.

In my view, then, the fat that we include in our diets needs to come from foods that provide a higher ratio of unsaturated to saturated fat. Or, very simply, another way of attacking the problem is to reduce or eliminate high-saturated fat content foods in our diets. (The saturated fat content of the following foods are in parenthesis.) Compare the following foods with the preceding chart to see how much saturated fat these food items put into your diet. Half-and-half (1 tbsp, 1.1 gram), whipping cream (1 tbsp, 3.5 grams), potato chips (10 chips, 2.1 grams), french fries (10 strips, 1.7 grams), cream cheese (1 ounce, 6.2 grams), Danish pastry (2 ounce, 4.7 grams), donut (2 ounce, 3.3 grams), milk chocolate bar (1 ounce, 5.5 grams), and one piece of apple pie (5 ounces, 3.9 grams).

Putting it another way, fruits, with the exception of avocados, would put zero grams of saturated fat into your diet.

How a 53-Year-Old Woman Lowered Blood Pressure and Cholesterol Level through Nutrition

A female patient, 53 years of age, had recently become a widow. On her last two office visits, I noticed a lowering of her energy level and that she had put on 20 pounds. She had a good job as chief bookkeeper for a large law firm and up to this time had always been energetic, and kept herself in trim. A physical examination showed basically an elevated blood pressure and nothing much else out of the ordinary. The blood cholesterol, however, was up also.

I discovered that she had gone on an eating binge—eating all of the pastries and rich foods that she had been careful to limit previously. She admitted that she didn't like to look in the mirror and was becoming indifferent to her appearance. As she unburdened herself of her grief, she came to the self-realization that she was actually adding to her problems. Because she was always a strongly motivated individual, it was not hard to convince her that she had to make diet alterations. In these cases, I need to add that my nurse, Betty, was always a staunch ally in explaining details of diets and answering the many questions that followed. We instructed the patient to cut way down on saturated fat foods and I also placed her on lecithin to see if that wouldn't also help with the cholesterol problem. She responded well and an office visit a few months later showed a fit and well-trimmed female. Both blood pressure and cholesterol came under control to normal levels.

Protein—Body Rejuvenators

Humans need an adequate source of protein in order to grow and replace tissue that wears out. Unlike fat, protein is not stored as reserve material in the body. While the body can draw upon certain tissue proteins, such as liver proteins, these supplies need replenishment to avoid the creation of a deficiency situation.

Proteins are the fundamental structural basis of all the cells of the body. In addition, certain proteins and protein derivatives are the functional elements in certain specialized cells, glandular secretions, enzymes, and hormones. As enzymes, proteins influence the breakdown of food for energy and the creation of new compounds for maintaining and repairing body tissue. Work, exercise, illness, and simple living activities exert a wear and tear on body tissue and proteins are the means by which the tissue is rebuilt. Because they are so vital in keeping the human body functioning, you should pay strict attention to the quality and quantity of proteins in your diet.

Amino Acids

Proteins consist of 22 or more nitrogen-containing compounds that are chemically referred to as amino acids. The amino acids are classified as: essential, partially essential, and nonessential. The essential amino acids, as the name suggests, are absolutely necessary for the body's functioning. They include:

leucine	tryptophan
isoleucine	valine
lysine	methionine
threonine	phenylalanine

The partly essential amino acids are: arginine, tyrosine, cystine, glycine, serine, and histidine.

The nonessential amino acids are: glutamic acid, aspartic acid, alanine, proline, and hydroxyproline.

At the beginning of this section, it was pointed out that arginine, one of the partly essential amino acids, has been found to play a role in stimulating the immune response. Thus, it would be wise to regard the classification of amino acids as being rather fluid. Again, we are at many frontiers in these areas and new discovery will cause shifts in the way these vital nutrient materials are regarded.

Generally speaking, animal proteins are of good biologic value, while most plant proteins are of fair to poor value. However, by eating a variety of the various protein foods, each containing some of the essential amino acids, you will in cumulative manner obtain all the necessary and essential amino acids.

The more essential amino acids a protein contains, the better it is for you. The animal proteins, such as meat, poultry, fish, eggs, milk (skim, dried, and whole), and milk products (cheese) are at the top of the list.

Plant products richest in protein include: soybeans, peanuts, cereals (especially wheat), peas, beans, and lentils.

A relative comparison of the protein value is contained in the following table. The "protein score" in the right-hand column endeavors to place a quantitative value on the amino acid content of each food listed.

milk (cow's)	78
egg	100
casein	80
egg albumin	100
beef muscle	83
beef liver	84
beef heart	80
beef kidney	77
pork tenderloin	86
fish	70
oats	79
rye	80
rice	72
corn meal	42
white flour	47
wheat germ	61
wheat gluten	40
soy flour	73
potato	56
navy bean	47
peas	58
sweet potato	81
spinach	70

The preceding is not a list from which you are to choose only the highest numbers. For example, while fish has a lower number than beef muscle, remember that the fat of fish is high in polyunsaturated, extra-long chain fatty acids. So, in this case, the trade-off has some positive effects if we elect to go with fish.

The rule, if there is any real dogma in this area, is to go for variety.

I recommend to my patients that one-third to one-half of the protein eaten daily be obtained from poultry, eggs, meat, or fish. It's important to space out the consumption of protein over all three meals. Too often I have found that my patients skip breakfast or eat only a donut or roll with a cup of coffee. Then, after a number of years of this kind of nutritional starvation, they wonder why they start to develop a host of physical problems—nerves, fatigue, sleeplessness, depression, and so on. As I have reiterated throughout the book, my first concern and job is to get them back on a sound and balanced eating pattern.

The Key Role of Minerals

Minerals are important to many vital living processes, both by themselves and in combination with each other. The amounts and ratios have to be accurately balanced and the human body does a magnificent job in adjusting the amounts that we provide and coming up with the right combinations.

One example of where balances are important is in the formation of bone where the amount and ratio of calcium to phosphorus is important. The recommended dietary intake for calcium has been established on the basis of an approximate one to one ratio with phosphorus.

For normal muscle functioning, the ratio between potassium and calcium in the fluid outside of the cells is important.

Sodium and potassium are the key factors in maintaining osmotic pressure, which regulates the passage or flow of water across semipermeable membranes throughout the body.

A number of minerals act as catalysts to control metabolic processes. Still others help make up certain organic compounds. For example, the hormone of the thyroid gland is a protein containing iodine. Iron is part of hemoglobin, zinc of insulin, cobalt of vitamin B-12, and sulfur is in biotin and thiamine.

The discovery of the importance of various minerals has been helped along by new analytical instrumentation and techniques. These include flame photometry, atomic absorption, and spectrophotometry. It is reasonable to assume that as even more advances are made in analysis, new and unknown roles will be discovered for existing minerals and others now residing in the trace mineral classification. New diagnostic equipment has been developed that rapidly analyzes minerals in the hair, serum, and urine and, which is important, in even smaller quantities than heretofore possible.

Calcium

Calcium is required by all the cells in the body. It is present in blood serum and has an important effect on nerve tissue. If the calcium level of the blood falls, the nervous system becomes hyperirritable. Thus, the glass of milk, which is rich in calcium, does indeed have a calming effect and helps induce restful sleep.

Calcium is necessary for blood clot formation because it acts as a catalyst in changing prothrombin to thrombin. It is also important in the rhythm of the heartbeat, in activating certain enzymes, and in controlling fluid flow through cell walls.

Calcium is necessary for bone formation and 99 percent of it is in the skeleton and teeth. When the diet furnishes an adequate intake of calcium, the bones serve as a storehouse for the mineral. This reserve is called on in times of stress to meet the body's increased need, in the event the diet is not supplying the correct amount.

Older people need to pay particular attention to obtaining adequate amounts of calcium to insure that bones retain their strength. Osteoporosis is characterized by demineralization of bone and is often associated with an inadequate calcium intake.

Research at the University of Chicago by Dr. Irwin Rosenberg has found that a corn sugar, known as glucose polymer, increases calcium absorption. A person absorbs an average of only one-third of the calcium consumed, and even less magnesium and zinc. This type research aimed at understanding and increasing absorption of nutrients helps us achieve the mineral balance required by our bodies.

Food sources include milk, dairy products except butter, green leafy vegetables, such as broccoli, kale, and turnip greens; and salmon, sardines, shrimp, and oysters. Because they contain oxalic acid that links up with calcium and reduces absorption, the exceptions in the green leafy vegetable group are spinach, beet greens, and chard. These foods are good for aiding the absorption of other nutrients like vitamin A, for example, but not for calcium.

Another factor to keep in mind in developing a diet to obtain adequate amounts of calcium—and this is important for women and older people—is that phosphorus compounds known as phytates can reduce calcium absorption. These are found in unrefined cereals.

The answer to the oxalate and phytate problem relative to obtaining enough calcium is to eat a variety of foods.

The recommended daily requirement for calcium is one gram for men and women.

Phosphorus

Phosphorus forms part of the bony structure and teeth where it is combined with calcium as calcium phosphate. Bone also has small amounts of carbonates, magnesium, sodium, and fluorine.

Phosphorus is a part of the compounds that determine the genetic code; DNA (deoxyribonucleic acid) and RNA (ribonucleic acid). It is also part of the energy-transporting systems in cells and phospholipids. Phospholipids take part in the emulsification or the forming of a suspension of fats and fatty acids and transporting these compounds in the suspended form. Phosphorus is needed by muscle in order to contract. It also assists in maintaining the acid-base balance of blood.

Sources of phosphorus include eggs, fish, poultry, meats, milk, cheese, beans, and nuts. The recommended daily requirement for phosphorus is one gram for both men and women.

Iron

The role of iron is closely intertwined with that of hemoglobin, which is the coloring material of the blood. Hemoglobin is a compound consisting of the protein, globin, and the iron-containing pigment, heme. Heme has the responsibility for transporting oxygen from the lungs to the tissues of the body. About 70 percent of the iron in the body is in the hemoglobin.

In addition, iron is found in muscle tissue and in cells as a part of enzymes. About 30 percent of the body's iron is stored in the liver, spleen, and bone marrow.

"Iron-poor blood" is more than an advertising slogan. It does happen that iron deficiency is the most prevalent nutritional deficiency occurring in humans. Illness, injury, surgery, or hemorrhage can be the causative factors behind an iron deficiency anemia. The anemia can also result very simply from a diet lacking a sufficient amount of iron or through faulty absorption of iron.

On the other hand, there is also the danger of iron overload. In the majority of cases this is a result of a genetic defect in which the body is unable to control iron absorption. If an anemia is diagnosed and iron supplementation is prescribed, it is important that a serum iron test be made to observe the course of the therapy. Symptoms of iron overload include cirrhosis of the liver, diabetes, and abnormal skin pigmentation. More information on iron and its importance to your health is provided in the next chapter.

Calf's liver is the best single source of dietary iron. In second place is beef liver. Other good sources of iron are kidney, heart, lean beef, oysters, and eggs. Green leafy vegetables are the best plant sources. Milk is a poor source of iron. The recommended daily allowance of iron is 18 mg.

I prescribe a chelated iron product for any of my patients experiencing an anemia. Because the iron that is available is not absorbed efficiently by the body, there are those of us who believe that by attaching iron to an organic compound the possibility of absorption is increased.

Sulfur

While sulfur is present in all cells of the body, it is most prevalent in the hair and nails. It is a part of insulin that regulates carbohydrate metabolism, thiamine (vitamin B-1), biotin, coenzyme A, which has been reported to be important in the formation of antibodies to fight infection, and in the anterior pituitary hormones. These hormones affect many other glands and their activity.

It is generally assumed that if the diet includes a sufficient amount of protein, the sulfur requirement will be met. Meat, fish, poultry, and eggs are principal sources.

Magnesium

Confusion, muscular tremor, nervous irritability, and dilation of the blood vessels are symptoms of magnesium deficiency. The tremor or tetany which is associated with a low blood level of magnesium is observed in alcoholism, diabetes, and parathyroid disease.

Magnesium is essential for cell formation and activates a number of enzyme systems related to the metabolism of phosphorus, carbohydrates, and protein. Magnesium has an important role as a coenzyme in protein synthesis.

Magnesium has an influence on tissue irritability and it has been shown that it is a central nervous system depressant. Thus, it acts to relax nerves.

Other experimental work on rats shows that high amounts of dietary magnesium seem to reduce fat deposits in blood vessels. More information on the healing power of magnesium is provided in the next chapter.

Sources of magnesium include nuts (almonds, brazil nuts, peanuts, cashews), molasses, shredded wheat, bran, wheat germ, watercress, soybean curd, chocolate, raw beet greens, fresh okra, spinach, and dates.

The requirement for magnesium is 400 mg. daily for adults.

Sodium, Potassium, and Chloride

Average diets usually contain sufficient amounts of sodium, potassium, and chloride to meet bodily needs. These chemical elements are involved in:

1. maintaining normal water balance and distribution
2. maintaining acid-base balance
3. maintaining normal muscular irritability

Sodium is the major factor involved in maintaining a proper water balance within the body and, also, functions in preserving the normal irritability of muscles. This simply means that muscles respond to nervous messages—in other words they do the work that is assigned to them. This can mean lifting, pushing, walking, etc. In addition to table salt (sodium chloride), many foods and food ingredients contain large amounts of sodium. These include beef, pork, cured meats, milk, cheese, eggs, baking powder, wheat breads, dill pickles, green olives, bouillon cubes, dry cereals, flavored gelatins, and canned vegetables.

Potassium is found mainly in the fluid inside of cells where it plays a role in cell metabolism, enzyme reactions, and the manufacture of muscle protein from amino acids in the blood. Potassium is necessary for muscular contraction and for nerve activity.

The use of certain diuretics and adrenal-cortical hormones may cause a depletion of potassium. Similarly, potassium losses may also occur as a result of vomiting and diarrhea.

Potassium is widely distributed in foods, including dairy products, fruits, vegetables, fish, nuts, and meat. Some comparisons may be of interest: one cup whole milk–370 mg., one cup buttermilk–1910 mg.; three ounces salmon–307 mg., three ounces sardines–502 mg.; one apple–152 mg., one avocado–1303 mg., one banana–440 mg., one-half canteloupe–682 mg., one cup fresh orange juice–496 mg., one slice watermelon–426 mg.; one cup asparagus–265 mg., one cup broccoli–414 mg., one cup collards–498 mg., one baked potato–556 mg., one cup winter squash–945 mg., and one tomato–300 mg.

Chloride is the negative ion most commonly associated with sodium in the fluid outside of body cells. To some extent, it is also found with potassium inside of the cells. Chloride aids in maintaining the acid-base balance in the body and the pressure that permits the passage of materials in and out of cells necessary for life's processes. During digestion some of the chloride is used for the manufacture of hydrochloric acid in the gastric glands and is subsequently secreted into the stomach.

Trace Elements

Copper. Copper is necessary for the utilization of iron in the manufacture of hemoglobin. It is also being found in an increasing number of enzymes and proteins. Copper may function in the formation of bone and in maintaining the sheath surrounding certain nerve fibers.

Humans do not generally fall prey to a deficiency of copper because of the small amounts that are required and its relative abundancy in foods. The human need is about two mg. daily. Foods containing copper include: liver, kidney, oysters, chocolate, nuts, cereals, raisins, molasses, and bone meal.

Cobalt. Cobalt is a constituent of vitamin B 12 and is evidently necessary for hemoglobin formation. It apparently aids iron absorption and functions in the synthesis of vitamin B-12 by bacteria in the intestinal tract. Only a small amount is necessary and the average diet is generally adequate. Cobalt is found in figs, cabbage, lettuce, spinach, beet greens, watercress, and buckwheat.

Iodine. As is well known, a lack of iodine in food and drinking water is related to the occurrence of simple goiters. In the absence of adequate iodine, the thyroid gland increases its secretory activity in an attempt to compensate for the deficiency and, as a result, the gland enlarges. The continuous use of iodized salt is necessary in low-iodine areas that are generally areas far from ocean water.

Iodine is an important part of the thyroid gland hormone, thyroxine, which maintains control of the energy metabolism of the body. Sufficient iodine must be supplied if that gland is to manufacture enough of the hormone thyroxine (T-4) and triiodothyroxine (T-3) to function normally.

The current requirement in human nutrition is 150 mcg. daily.

There are certain substances that tend to produce goiters and are known as goitrogens. It has been demonstrated that such a substance is found in vegetables. An excessive consumption of cabbage, cauliflower, Brussels sprouts, and peanuts can possibly lead to the development of a goiterous condition.

Sources of iodine include oysters, sardines, clams, lobsters, and other seafoods.

Zinc. Dwarfism, lack of development of secondary sexual characteristics in the male, and iron-deficiency anemia have been found in populations where zinc intake is inadequate. Hypogeusia, or a lack of taste sensation, is another symptom of a shortage of zinc in the diet. It is also important in burn and wound healing, and carbohydrate digestion. Zinc seems to be present in the pancreas and it accompanies insulin when this hormone is manufactured. There is also evidence that zinc is important in protein utilization.

There are a number of diseases in which zinc levels are below normal, including bronchitis, pyelonephritis (a kidney infection), and pneumonia. Decreased zinc levels have also been associated with myocardial infarctions (heart attacks), various types of cancer, alcoholism, liver disease, rheumatoid arthritis, and inflammatory bowel disease. In reporting this information, the implication is not intended that zinc supplementation will arrest or ameliorate the conditions but to indicate the lines of research and information that have been produced. The understanding and importance of zinc in physiological processes is growing significantly and it would certainly be prudent for anyone taking a multivitamin and mineral preparation to be sure that zinc is included among the minerals.

An immunologist and director of cancer research at the Oklahoma Medical Research Foundation, Dr. Robert Good, is reported to have said that zinc deficiency in older people may make them more susceptible to many diseases, including cancer.

Personally, I think that the availability of zinc and other nutrients in our food sources may not be as great a problem as is absorption for older people. For that reason and for a long time, I have tended to use chelated minerals that involve attaching the minerals to amino acids or other organic compounds to aid absorption of the mineral by the body.

Prostate Problem Relieved with My Nutritional Therapy

A patient of mine referred her husband to me because of an intermittent prostate problem. He had been to a urologist who recommended surgery. Wanting to explore alternative therapies, he came to me because of his wife's knowledge of my nutritional interests.

An examination showed the prostate to be enlarged and somewhat tender. There appeared to be no nodules. There was a history of frequent need to urinate during sleep hours. The patient's diet turned out to consist of a large percentage of high-saturated fat foods, including snack foods, ice cream, cookies, pastries, and candy. I learned that while his wife prepared nutritious meals at home, he fell off the nutritional wagon at work with access to the mentioned foods in dispensing machines in the plant lunch room. During breaks and at lunch, he loaded up on high-fat foods because, as he said, "I'm a pipefitter, I work outside a lot, and I need the energy." I learned, too, that he liked to stop after work to have a few beers before going home. His whole dietary program, as I saw it, was robbing his body of valuable nutrients, including important zinc.

I said to him that possibly something could be done about the prostate problem but that it would take a pretty thorough reorientation of his eating patterns. He agreed and we made certain that he understood the high-saturated fat foods would have to be eliminated. There has been some evidence implicating fat and cholesterol with prostate problems.

I told him that I was going to have my nurse call his wife and make suggestions about the lunches he took to work. To help him with his need for snacks, we recommended that she put in such high-zinc sources as sunflower seeds, soybean nuts, and other nuts. Since he had a refrigerator at work in which he could put his lunch, we suggested that she occasionally include a carton of yogurt or cottage cheese. For his breakfasts, we suggested that he sprinkle wheat germ on his cereals for an added source of zinc. For dinners we suggested liver, shellfish, poultry, and beef. I also prescribed a chelated zinc tablet and a multivitamin and mineral preparation, and suggested that the beer after work be scaled down.

On subsequent office visits by his wife, she reported that he was sticking to the new dietary regime. He came in for a scheduled office visit in three months and he said that the frequency of urination had subsided. An examination showed a decrease in the swelling of the prostate. He came in again a few months later and it appeared as though the swelling had subsided even more and that he was having few to little problems with the condition. He was grateful that he was able to find an alternative to surgery. Before embarking on such therapy, prostate sufferers should have thorough physical examinations and be in consultation with a nutritionally competent physician who can determine possible success for this route and guide the patient accordingly.

Sources of zinc include shellfish, meat, poultry, cheese, whole grain cereals,, dry beans, cocoa, and nuts. The recommended daily intake for adults is 15 mg.

Other trace elements include:

Chromium. Chromium activates several enzymes involved in the manufacture of fatty acids and cholesterol. It appears to inhibit the formation of aortic plaques or plates, and a deficiency of chromium may contribute to atherosclerosis. It also appears to be associated with the ability of the body to use glucose and thus may influence the development of hypoglycemia. It is also linked with the transport of amino acids into cells. Sources are brewer's yeast, liver, corn oil, whole grain cereals, and beef.

Molybdenum. It is a constituent of certain enzymes and may help in the utilization of iron. It is found in liver, kidney, leafy vegetables, whole grains, peas, and beans.

Selenium. Within the last few years, selenium has joined the ranks of essential trace minerals. Animal experiments show it effectively replaces vitamin E where animals had diets lacking in vitamin E. It is thought that selenium may be beneficial in preventing heart disease and cancer. Food sources include liver, kidney, heart, whole grains, vegetables, tuna, and herring. See next chapter for a more complete discussion of selenium.

Chapter 5

Important Nutritional Discoveries Involving Selenium, Magnesium, and Iron

Selenium—Emerging from the Wings to Take on Anti-Cancer and Cardiac Health Roles

Selenium is a mineral that has been emerging, you might say, from the wings of the nutritional theater. It has not been on center stage because very little of it is needed, normally in the microgram range, and because its reputation has been tainted as a toxic material. This is due to the fact that it is similar chemically to sulfur and can replace sulfur in the structure of a number of key enzymes. When this occurs the enzymes are not able to carry out their functions in the body and the resulting symptoms can lead to death. The symptoms of selenium toxicity include appetite loss, hair loss, progressive paralysis, and spinal column pain and weakness.

Continuing research has identified the fact that it is selenium in its inorganic forms that are the dangerous performers. These include sodium selenite and various selenium salts and acids. On the other hand, when nutritional selenium is made available in association with organic amino acids, it is able to perform a beneficial role.

A toxic dose of selenium is estimated to be at least ten times the amount which might be used in a therapeutic situation. Therapeutic, or beneficial, and toxic, or harmful, amounts vary in everything that we ingest, whether it is apples, heart drugs, salt, beer, water, peanuts, or what have you. Careful monitoring of the therapeutic dose of any nutrient material under the guidance of a nutritionally-oriented medical professional is necessary.

One of the other problems in recognizing the nutritional importance of selenium in health maintenance and in therapy is its rather scarce presence in the soil. Some land has it in relative abundance and other growing areas have been severely leached of the selenium content. It has taken a while to identify these regions and then to demonstrate what its presence or absence has meant, if anything, to living things. The work that has been done has centered principally on livestock and, subsequently, the data have been shown to have applicability to humans as well. At the end of this chapter, I am going to recount my own rather recent experience in treating a cardiac condition with selenium.

Research has identified liver necrosis, abnormal heart function, high blood pressure, infertility, and a muscular dystrophy disease, among others, as due to selenium deficiency in some 40 types of farm animals. Cattle farmers in Ohio, where the soil is selenium deficient, buy grain from South Dakota where the soil is rich in selenium. They do this to avoid their cattle developing "white muscle disease."

How Selenium Can Prevent the Spread of Cancer

It has been shown that selenium can prevent the spread of some existing tumors and block the taking hold of transplanted tumors in laboratory animals.

In New Zealand selenium was added to feed and to washing solutions that are used to control insects on sheep. This move was credited with eliminating certain forms of cancer in sheep in the country. The soil in New Zealand is selenium poor.

In one research study, a strain of mice that usually develops mammary cancer at an 82 percent rate was shown to drop to a 10 percent rate when selenium was added to the feed.

This effect of selenium seems to be corroborated in humans. In Japan, where the soil is rich in selenium, the death rate from breast cancer is lower than in the U.S., which on a relative scale has selenium-poor soil. The same situation prevails with respect to lung cancer—an average of 13 cases per 100,000 population in Japan as opposed to 37 cases per 100,000 in the U.S. It is reported that the average intake of selenium in Japan is 200 to 300 micrograms daily compared to 60 to 100 micrograms in the American diet.

Looking at colon cancer, studies claim about three deaths per 100,000 population in Venezuela which has a relatively high selenium content in its soil. This contrasts with approximately 14 deaths per 100,000 in the U.S. from colon cancer. Milk is reported to have up to ten times more selenium in Venezuela than milk produced in certain regions of the U.S.

Data apparently show the U.S. to be at or near the bottom in selenium consumption on a per person basis. The selenium blood level in individuals in such countries as Japan, Taiwan, and Thailand is reported as 0.20 parts per million. In the U.S., however, the average is 0.07 parts per million. This average also applies to such countries as the United Kingdom, New Zealand, and Australia.

How Does It Carry Out Its Anti-Cancer Role?

Selenium is a scavenger of "free radicals" in the body. These are molecular bits and pieces remaining from incomplete metabolic oxidation of fats and proteins. They are sometimes called peroxides. They are potentially harmful because they attach themselves to normal molecules and take away vital components. In this manner they destroy the cell's ability to function at top performance. Some research has shown the free radicals to have cancer-causing properties.

There is an enzyme called glutathione peroxidase that can attach itself to free radicals, and in the process, renders them inactive. This, then, protects normal cells from the free radicals. Selenium is an integral part of the enzyme.

Another apparent action of selenium is its ability to scavenge carcinogenic materials such as nitrosamines and polychlorobiphenyls or PCBs. PCBs have been in the news lately and have been used in various types of electrical equipment. When discarded the equipment poses dangers because of the possibility of the polychlorobiphenyls being released and leaching into underground water supplies. Selenium, also, apparently has the ability to take up such dangerous metals as cadmium and mercury, and unburned hydrocarbons (smog).

Another important function of selenium that is exciting to me is its ability to aid the body's own immune system. Researchers have shown that selenium is a key to the formation of antibodies and ubiquinone (coenzyme Q) which protects against both infectious diseases and malignancies. Veterinary studies have shown this to be true in livestock, especially in protecting newly born chicks from infection. Other research with mice has shown selenium to play an important part in the activity of phagocytes—the white blood cells that attack foreign invaders of our bodies.

Selenium's Role in Combating Heart Problems

Wilfred E. Shute, a Canadian physician who has long pioneered the use of vitamin E in treating heart problems, states that selenium and vitamin E work well as a pair. The one nutrient aids and improves the effect of the other and vice versa. The result is that less of each nutrient is needed than when either is used alone.

Selenium and vitamin E benefit the heart because they improve oxygen utilization in the cells. And, this comes from their ability to scavenge the free radicals that were mentioned earlier in this chapter. This action allows the cells to function more efficiently and with less oxygen demand.

Other work shows that selenium is important in biochemical processes that aid the construction of the blood vessel network in tissues, particularly the heart and lungs. In addition to reducing oxygen need at the cell and tissue level, selenium in combination with vitamin E provides an improved delivery of oxygen by helping form an excellent foundation of veins and arteries.

My Own Experience with Selenium Treatment

I have been bothered with extra systoles of the heart, which simply means that instead of, if we can relate this to a clock, a steady tick-tock type of rhythm, there is a rapid tick, tick, tick, and then a tock type of rhythm. It probably started with me when, after performing surgery, I would drink a few cups of strong coffee to pick up my energies. It picked me up but, unfortunately, it jolted my heart muscle into this irregular pattern that has remained with me. I have been taking a prescription drug prescribed by my cardiologist to control this condition. Some months ago I noted a reference to selenium's ability to aid heart problems. I placed myself on a therapeutic dose of organically complexed selenium to see what might occur. I was more than pleasantly surprised to note that this therapy controlled the extra systoles and in consultation with my cardiologist, I reduced the heart prescription. I, of course, take vitamin E as a regular supplement and I believe that the combination of the two have greatly aided me.

How Selenium May Help Other Conditions

There is some work that shows that selenium apparently can help maintain light receptors in the retina of the eye, in addition to aiding the building of a blood vessel network in the retina. As a sidelight to this clinical observation by one physician, it was reported that some patients obtained relief from arthritis and diabetes symptoms. Whether directly related to the action of selenium is open to question.

There is other work that relates a deficiency of selenium in the diet to male sterility, hypertension, a susceptibility to heavy metal poisoning, improper breakdown of protein in the body, and poor hair and skin tone. It will be noted, for example, that selenium sulfide is listed as an ingredient of a number of shampoos that are used to control dandruff.

Availability of Selenium

Because the United States, as mentioned at the beginning of the chapter, has soil that is relatively poor in selenium, the possibility of obtaining therapeutic amounts of selenium from fruit and vegetable sources is not great. In addition, synthetic fertilizers that are often high in sulfur content contribute to selenium deficiency in the soil, because sulfur and selenium are biochemically antagonistic to each other.

It appears that selenium supplements are one of the few available ways of obtaining therapeutic amounts of the mineral. The supplements are derived from yeast that has been grown in a selenium-concentrated medium. In addition, I should point out that the action of selenium is aided by also including such established antioxidants as vitamins A, C, and E in the formulation of such supplements.

How Magnesium Relieves Nervous Tension

I would like to mention two cases that presented symptoms of involuntary muscle movement or tics. The first was a female patient, 65 years of age, who had an involuntary movement of the upper-right eyelid. This is, of course, a disconcerting type of affliction because people to whom you are talking have a tendency to have their gaze focus on the involuntary movement. In turn, this makes the patient even more self-conscious and can cause even more prolonged movement. This patient has gone to one of the leading clinics of the country and after a thorough examination and many diagnostic tests, the recommendation was that it would be necessary to sever the nerve that controls the movement of the eyelid. She did not immediately follow this recommendation and came to me for a gynecological examination, after having been referred to me by another doctor. During the course of the history taking, she volunteered the information regarding her eyelid. I asked her if she would be willing to try a simple treatment for the condition. She agreed and I prescribed chelated magnesium. After taking the chelated magnesium orally for approximately four weeks, she regained complete control of the eyelid. I saw her one year after the treatment was first started and she reported that she had no recurrence of the problem and was very pleased that she had not gone ahead with the operation.

The second case involved a female patient, 45 years of age, who came in for a periodic gynecological examination.

During the history-taking process, she mentioned that she had been in a hospital for two weeks for a neurological examination. She was having problems with involuntary movement of her head. I asked her what the outcomes of the neurological tests were and she replied that all of them were negative. Thereupon, I suggested that we might try magnesium for these movements. She stated that she was willing to try and I prescribed chelated magnesium. A few weeks later she returned to the office for the results of the gynecological tests and was elated that the head movements were now under control.

A Natural Tranquilizer

In my practice I have found magnesium helpful to patients with two other types of problems. The first involves patients who have a problem resting or going to sleep at night, and closely associated with them are those people who are constantly on edge, who are nervous and high strung.

A typical case belonging to the first group is that of a female, 70 years of age, who is a writer and active in all aspects of her life—whether writing a story or baking a cake. She came in reporting that she was having trouble sleeping at night and was taking sleeping pills that had helped at first but were now useless. While she was not a heavy coffee drinker, I did convince her to cut down her caffeine consumption in order to minimize that stimulating effect. Finally, I asked her to try chelated magnesium and after a course of therapy lasting one month, she came back remarking how well it had worked for her. As we might expect she reported being able to approach her writing projects and assignments with more energy and staying power. She said that she was able to sleep longer than she ever had and without taking anything in the way of sleeping pills.

I have been able to help many nervous and high-strung females achieve a new feeling of tranquility through the use of magnesium. As far as age is concerned, they range from teenagers to the postmenopausal group. While I mention female patients, this is only because I am an obstetrician-gynecologist. The therapy that I mention here should work equally well for men.

A typical case is that of a young lady, 24 years of age, who was under considerable strain in her position as secretary to a very demanding attorney. She had a substantial amount of responsibility, and when she left the office in the evening, she said that she was completely drained. She said that she was able to survive the day only by consuming large amounts of coffee and cola drinks. The result was that she was very nervous and emotional and, of course, the coffee with its caffeine content was simply compounding the problem. Rather than have her give up all types of refreshment during the day, I convined her to start drinking decaffeinated coffee and soft drinks. I put her on a course of chelated magnesium therapy and within two months, she reported that she was handling the pressures much better and that her co-workers commented that she appeared to be more relaxed. The biggest benefit, she said, was that it did not take her the entire evening to wind down from the day's work.

Relief of Muscle Strain

In addition to exerting a tranquilizing effect, magnesium in combination with calcium has a positive effect on muscle and soft tissue strain and injury. These include backaches, stiff necks, sore joints, and muscle spasms brought on by too strenuous physical work or exercise.

Iron—How to Combat Anemia

Anemia is a medical problem in which the amount of hemoglobin or the number of red blood cells is below normal. Iron-deficiency anemia is referred to as the most common of nutritional deficiencies.

The reasons for the iron deficiency can include chronic blood loss, defective absorption, inadequate amounts of iron in the diet, or increased requirement as in growth or pregnancy. Chronic blood loss can go unrecognized. For example, the excessive use of aspirin or alcoholism can result in chronic blood loss. Other sources of bleeding may be hemorrhoids, gastric ulcer, or colitis. In treating the problem of iron deficiency, it is important to diagnose and treat the causes of blood loss.

Iron is a necessary part of hemoglobin, which is composed of protein, globin, and the iron-containing pigment, heme. Heme is responsible for the oxygen-carrying capacity of blood.

With this brief introduction to hemoglobin, it is easier to understand the symptoms of iron-deficiency anemia. These include lack of endurance, shortness of breath on exertion, constant tiredness, and palpitation or consciousness of a pounding heartbeat. I observe a pallor to the skin, coldness of hands and feet, and fingernails are lusterless, thin, and brittle.

Because of my specialty of obstetrics and gynecology, I, perhaps, see more cases of iron-deficiency anemias than other physicians. The menstrual cycle and pregnancy require more attention to iron in the diet. Above and beyond that, however, is what I believe is a strong precipitating factor—high-carbohydrate, low-protein eating patterns. Long-term improvement in the condition, obviously, requires long-term diet alteration.

My Anemia Therapy

My therapeutic approach stresses iron supplementation and a high-protein diet. Because beef liver is high in both iron and protein, I recommend it at least once a week. For example, a typical three ounce serving of beef liver furnishes 7.5 mg. of iron and 22 grams of protein.

I stress other meat sources because they have a greater part of the iron in the organic or heme form which can be absorbed more readily.

Iron needs to dissolve in hydrochloric acid in the stomach in order to be absorbed effectively. Acid-containing foods such as citrus juices, fruits, yogurt, and buttermilk can assist in iron absorption. Ascorbic acid (vitamin C) can aid iron absorption.

In addition to liver, other good sources of iron include:

sardines (3 ounces)	2.5 mg.
shrimp (3 ounces)	2.6 mg.
beef (3 ounces)	2.7 mg.
steak (3 ounces)	2.5 mg.
beef heart (3 ounces)	5.0 mg.
veal (3 ounces)	2.7 mg.
apricots (4 ounces, dried, uncooked)	3.6 mg.
dates (10, whole)	2.4 mg.
raisins (one ounce packet)	1.0 mg.
whole wheat bread (one slice)	0.8 mg.
sunflower seeds (4 ounces)	5.1 mg.
beans, lima (4 ounces)	2.3 mg.
broccoli (one stalk)	1.4 mg.
kale (one cup, raw)	1.8 mg.
lettuce (wedge, ¼ head)	0.7 mg.
egg yolk (one)	0.9 mg.

Sources estimate the daily requirements of iron for adult men at 0.65 to 1.3 mg., menstruating women at 0.7 to 2.3 mg., adolescent girls at 1 to 2.7 mg., and adolescent boys at 1 to 2 mg. With a recommended daily allowance of 18 mg. and allowing for a ten percent rate of absorption, the adult male's need is met—1.8 mg. is greater than the upper limit of 1.3 mg. However, when we look at the upper limit for menstruating women of 2.3 mg. maturing girls of 2.7 mg., and maturing boys of 2 mg., the 1.8 mg. falls short. On this basis this group might reasonably look to increase their intake above the 18 mg. level to meet their increased needs. The need is based on what has been worked out to be average daily attrition or loss of iron from the body.

Thus, when I am faced with an iron-deficiency anemia, I need to consider not only the deficiency but, also, what normal losses occur. This is why there must be diet correction, in addition to supplementation with iron sources.

Before citing a few cases, I want to mention a habit that can lead to iron deficiency and that is the overuse of antacid preparations. As was mentioned, the acid in the stomach assists the absorption of iron. Thus, when the acidity is neutralized by antacids, the iron goes through the intestinal tract and is eliminated without absorption. Readers who have the habit of using antacids should keep this in mind relative to obtaining the benefit of the iron in their diets.

Also keep in mind the earlier recommendation in this book about not overcooking vegetables. You not only lose iron but, also, other minerals and vitamins that these valuable food sources contain. Vegetables cooked too long or at too high a temperature are virtually without mineral and vitamin value.

How Simple Dietary Changes Cure Anemia: Three Cases

The patient was a 40-year-old woman who had bouts of extreme fatigue, dizziness, and weakness. She was listless and had a grey pallor to her skin. She said that it had started a couple of years back and had gotten progressively worse to the point where she just dragged around the house. Her husband had lost interest in her sexually which compounded the problem.

Talking about the kind of diet she followed, I learned that it consisted almost entirely of carbohydrates. We provided her with a diet plan that emphasized liver at least twice a week in the early stages, along with beef roasts, steaks, and stews as they could be worked in. I also emphasized raw, green leafy vegetables—at least two each day. For her sweet tooth, I advised that she nibble on dried raisins or apricots during the day. These dried fruits are excellent iron sources.

Once I was satisfied that she had a good foundation in her eating habits, I prescribed a chelated iron tablet and a multi-vitamin and mineral supplement. The chelated iron is my own special preference because I believe that the absorption of iron is assisted. Within six weeks she reported that she was feeling better and the tests that we did confirmed an upsurge in iron in her system. Because this was a longstanding condition, I advised that she continue with the general dietary program with, perhaps, a reduction of the liver to once a week. In cases of this kind, there is a tendency to stop the treatment recommendations just as soon as the first sign of improvement is noted. This is a mistake. It is important to check with your physician, so that the condition can be monitored.

Another case was that of a 26-year-old woman who received the same evaluation and dietary program but who showed no apparent improvement with the chelated iron supplementation. Neither the hematocrit (ratio of packed red blood cells to the volume of whole blood) nor the hemoglobin values improved.

In this case I added the use of folic acid, one mg. three times daily. This additional supplement had a positive effect and her condition improved.

Another case was that of a 35-year-old woman, who like the previous individual, was not aided by the iron supplementation. In this case I tried a combination of vitamin E and iron. In this particular case, the combination resulted in a reversal of the iron-deficiency anemia.

There have been studies that indicate that vitamin E plays a role in combating certain human nutritional anemias. Other evidence shows that alpha tocopherol, which is part of the vitamin E complex, may be involved in the production of the heme portion of hemoglobin.

There are other types of anemia besides the kind resulting from a deficiency of iron. These cannot be handled alone through dietary or nutritional means. Your physician should be the one to diagnose and treat these other types of anemia. Actually, whenever there are symptoms as were cited, do not attempt to treat yourself right away. First, go to a nutritionally competent physician, have the diagnostic tests done, and then see if the condition is due to an iron deficiency.

In the meantime, be aware of how iron losses can occur, such as overcooked vegetables, or the excessive use of antacids for upset stomachs.

Be aware that we require protein in our diets and that meat sources provide a superior source of iron. Avoid loading your diet with too many carbohydrates because you will be robbing your body of the iron necessary for the proper functioning of the blood in your vascular system.

Chapter 6

Your Body's Catalysts and Wonder Chemicals—How to Benefit from Them

The world's best chemical engineers could not design and construct as technologically remarkable a manufacturing process as that which occurs in our bodies and sees raw materials (food) of varying quantity and quality converted by thousands of chemical reactions into products necessary to power the cells in our bodies. In fact, the manufacturing process is so complex that biochemists will be doing their research work for decades to come trying to unravel the chemical reactions occurring and the compounds involved.

The Accelerators

Catalysts are substances that speed up or accelerate chemical reactions. They are used in all kinds of chemical plant operations. Enzymes are the catalysts, or accelerators, in our bodies. They are there to speed up such physiological processes as vision, breathing, storage and release of energy, transmission of nerve impulses, muscle contraction, reproduction process, and, of course, the digestion of food. We mentioned that there are thousands of chemical reactions occurring and it is estimated that there are three to five times as many enzymes. Putting it another way, for each chemical reaction to be carried out, three to five enzymes are necessary. To date, some sources state that only 1000 have been identified.

Enzymes are interesting since they are specific in their roles. While some enzymes are involved with such diverse functions as muscle contraction and nerve pulse transmission, we, since we're concerned with nutrition, will concentrate on those that aid in breaking down fats, digesting carbohydrates, and working with protein. These jobs are accomplished exceedingly fast; some, for example, can perform their functions a million or more times a minute.

Enzymes are protein molecules that are produced by the cells. While some enzymes consist only of protein, others have a nonprotein portion without which they cannot function. The nonprotein part in some cases is a trace element such as zinc, magnesium, manganese, or molybdenum; in other cases it may be a vitamin-related structure; finally, in still other instances, the enzymes may contain both the trace element and the vitamin-related compound.

The Role of Enzymes in Digestion

Manufacturing processes in chemical plants require as uniform a raw material as possible in order to process it into a satisfactory end product. If it is "off specifications," it can play havoc with subsequent processing steps. Some equipment, for example, may be set to operate at a certain temperature or pressure to carry out a reaction. The "off spec" raw material may not work at this temperature and cause poor product and yield, equipment outages, and other problems.

Now, let us compare this to the chemical manufacturing process occurring in our bodies. Hopefully, we supply our bodies with good quality raw material, in the form of food, which then can be reacted to and processed satisfactorily to the end products necessary for our cells to function. In this regard we are lucky, indeed, that we have enzymes to accelerate the chemical reactions involved in food digestion. Their presence often makes up for some of the "off spec" material that we send down to our stomachs. Sometimes, however, we pay the price for some of our eating indiscretions and even the enzymes cannot carry out their magic. Stomach upset, nausea, gas, and even more toxic reactions may occur.

While food digestion begins as a mechanical process in the mouth with grinding, tearing, and crushing action of the teeth, the main action is performed by enzymes. Amylases are enzymes in the secretions of the salivary and pancreatic glands that are important in the breakdown of carbohydrates. Lipase is another enzyme from the pancreas and it accelerates the digestion of fat. Sucrase from the small intestine acts on sugar, or sucrose, to convert it into glucose and fructose. Pepsin in the stomach aids the digestion of protein that is acted upon further by a pancreatic enzyme, trypsin, and intestinal enzymes, the peptidases.

Obviously, the preceding only touches upon the hundreds and hundreds of steps and reactions that occur when food is broken down into the nutrient materials which can be absorbed and utilized by cells. And, the reactions are speeded along by the wonderful enzyme system. If they did not hurry things along, we wouldn't have room for each succeeding meal.

Inborn Errors of Metabolism

I think it's important to bear in mind that heredity plays an important role in whether we have all of the thousands of enzymes we should have. In the event we have problems digesting certain foods, it may very well be that there is a missing enzyme or one in short supply. Enzymes are structured and regulated by genes and problems with the controlling genes can produce a deficiency or impaired functioning of enzymes that can be transmitted from generation to generation. The full impact of these occurrences is that some authorities believe that inherited disorders of metabolism are the single most common cause of disease in human beings.

An example of a rather well-known disease caused by an enzyme deficiency is phenylketonuria (PKU). This disease results from a defect in the formation of an enzyme necessary to break down the substance phenylalanine. Unless detected in the newborn, mental retardation results. Tests for PKU are done routinely on newborn infants in most hospitals. Treatment consists of diets low in phenylalanine, and a proprietary formula has been developed for this purpose.

There are four ways in which inherited errors can be handled:

1. Minimizing the intake of the nutrient material that cannot be handled satisfactorily, such as in the case of PKU.
2. Predigesting the troublesome, or as in some cases, toxic, nutrient. An example of this is fermentation of lactose-containing milks in case of deficiency of the enzyme lactase, or hydrolysis of protein in the case of trypsinogen lack.
3. A third way of handling an inborn error in the enzyme system is to try to enhance enzyme activity. This depends on whether or not there is some enzyme activity to begin with. In the event there is, it may be possible to stimulate the production of the enzyme by introducing extra amounts of the nonprotein portions that were mentioned earlier in this chapter. These are the trace elements and vitamins necessary to make the enzyme a functioning whole.
4. A fourth way is to supply the enzyme directly, if it is available. For example, pepsin, trypsin, peptidases, and lipase, to name a few, are available. Children who have cystic fibrosis are helped by having intestinal enzymes provided directly.

Aiding Our Enzymes

Even if we are fortunate enough not to have a hereditary defect in our enzyme systems, all of us are probably deficient in this area. The degree to which we might be deficient can vary according to a number of factors, such as age, occupational stress, environment, sex, disease conditions, and diet. Of these factors, there is only one that we can do much about and that is diet. Since we can't grow younger, probably cannot quickly change our jobs, nor can we immediately change things in the environment such as noise and air pollution, probably all we can change is our diet.

Steps You Can Take to Boost Your Enzyme Performance

1. As we mentioned, some enzymes cannot function without the nonprotein portions being present. The nonprotein portion comes from trace elements such as zinc, manganese, molybdenum, copper, and magnesium, and from various vitamins. Eat from a wide variety of food sources as mentioned repeatedly throughout this book to provide your nutritional base. Use a broad-spectrum vitamin-mineral supplement to add insurance that your enzyme system will have the necessary raw materials. By using a broad-spectrum approach, each newly discovered importance of this mineral or vitamin to our health and enzyme systems need not overly concern you. You, undoubtedly, will have included them in your well-planned and diverse nutritional program.

2. Provide your body with the highest quality raw material in the form of food that you can. By doing so you will give the enzyme system an opportunity to do its job efficiently. Under most circumstances, you will probably find that a piece of whole wheat toast is far easier to digest than a donut made with a saturated oil or an apple versus a piece of whipped cream pie. The high-quality foods are the vegetables, fruits, poultry, fish and so forth versus the snack foods, cookies, hot dogs, and sausages. Just as in a chemical plant, high-quality raw materials mean high-quality end products.

3. Again, in a comparison between chemical plants and our bodies, most 30- or 40-year-old chemical plants are ready for phase out.

The remarkable chemical manufacturing systems in our bodies, however, after 30 or 40 years are good for another 30 or 40 years of service if we practice good preventive maintenance. The most important aspect of preventive maintenance in this instance is moderation.

Don't load up on foods to the point of discomfort. At that particular point, your digestive system, including the enzymes, is telling you that you are exceeding the capacity of your processing machinery.

Don't wear out your enzyme sytem by overindulgence in food and drink and it will allow you to enjoy the same foods in your later years as those that gave you pleasure when you were young.

I think that osteoporosis, which afflicts so many of the aged, may not be due to a lack of calcium in the diet but rather to an inability of the enzyme system to process it. In cases of this kind, enzyme therapy may be necessary.

Hydrogen Oxide— The Oldest and Cheapest Wonder Drug

This is the Age of Wonder Woman, Bionic Man, Wonder Antibiotics, Wonder Drugs, and Wonder Chemicals. It is true that medical science has made tremendous advances as a result of new drug discoveries capable of knocking out infections and curing or relieving the symptoms of a host of diseases. On the other hand, we have to temper our admiration for these discoveries because the pharmaceutical preparations, including the antibiotics, can be dangerous if not administered or prescribed properly. The drugs are wonderful but there can be side effects and care must be exercised in their use by the physician.

Out of all of these wonder drugs, there is one that has been around for a very long time—in fact, since time began on earth. In contrast to the other drugs, it probably should be used more often. It's relatively safe in its pure form, very valuable in its beneficial effect and still quite inexpensive. No prescription is required from a physician and it's much better than a lot of other chemicals around for what it can do.

This wonder drug, or chemical, is hydrogen oxide.

Its chemical formula is H_2O, or just plain water.

Of course, with some of the treatments it receives, it's probably not correct to refer to it as *just plain* water. Of course, there is a way out of this because there are many spring and distilled waters available.

In medicine, I think we have become so dazzled by the spectacular and sophisticated electronic gadgetry, scanners, and diagnostic machines that we forget to emphasize and impart some fundamental and basic nutritional advice to our patients. One of these is that water, again in its pure form, is a very vital and important adjunct to good health.

Then, too, in the world of food, we consumers have had thrust upon us several score substitutes for just plain water. From the ubiquitous vending machines pour billions of cans of soft drinks. These are colored and flavored water with sugar or sugar substitutes added and are far less valuable to humans than plain water. Also substituting for water are coffee, tea, fruit drinks, fruit juices (often sweetened to excess), beer, wine, and alcoholic drinks.

Milk is a fairly good substitute for water but it does not quite have the solubilizing effect that water does—particularly after a heavy meal has been eaten. A glass of water has a clean taste and cleansing effect on the mouth and teeth.

It is my observation with patients that they drink far less water than they should. One glass seems to be about average and it's rare to find a patient admitting to drinking two glasses of water daily. The importance of drinking water is simply not emphasized anywhere in our daily lives—not by newspapers, television, doctors, or medical groups or societies.

The Food and Nutrition Board recommends one milliliter of water per calorie of food. This is for all healthy individuals except infants. Thus, if a diet consists of about 2500 calories per day, then there is a need according to this recommendation for 2500 ml., or 2.5 liters, of water. This is slightly over 2.5 quarts of water or about ten glasses. Most people obtain part of this requirement through juices, milk, soup, vegetables, fruits, and other sources. My recommendation, then, is that you drink four to five glasses of water daily.

The Importance of Water

An excessive intake of salt or other minerals, or a high-protein diet, increases the need for liquid to aid in the elimination of waste. It is important that salt, for example, not be allowed to reach too high a concentration in the body. It can have a toxic effect, as it upsets electrolytic balances throughout the body and, particularly, the kidneys. Fortunately, a thirst mechanism asserts itself, in the event an individual has been munching on potato chips, popcorn, or peanuts, and the body craves a liquid. The tavern owner is aware of this, of course, when he provides bowls of salty popcorn and peanuts in order to stimulate the thirst mechanism and increase the volume of beer and other alcoholic beverages consumed by his patrons.

The intake of concentrated sweets, also, stimulates the need for water in order to dilute the effect of the sugars. Many people, after a sundae or malt, crave water to dilute or dissipate the heavy feeling that is often an accompanying effect. In addition, some people will thirst for water to wash away the sweet and cloying effect from their mouths after ice cream, candy, or other sweets are consumed.

While gastric juices perform well in handling the food substances we send to the stomach, we can make the job still easier by providing the universal solvent, water. Carbohydrates, proteins, and fats require a molecule of water for each amino acid molecule or pair of sugar molecules that split off.

A Transport Medium for Vital Nutrients

Water acts as a transport medium for vitamins, minerals, and other nutrients to where they are needed by the body.

A Temperature Regulator

Water helps regulate the temperature of the body. Water is lost in the form of sweat to remove heat and help maintain the 98.6 degrees temperature which is the optimum temperature for the operation of our various biological systems.

The Natural Aid to Regularity

Not only does water carry valuable nutrients throughout the body but, also, it helps remove waste products through the kidneys and bowels.

Water in the intestinal tract aids elimination and promotes regularity by softening the feces. Limiting the intake of water, on the other hand, tends to make the feces dry and hard. And, it is my opinion, that hemorrhoids can be prevented by a good percentage of those afflicted with the condition, if these people drink sufficient quantities of water. Soft stools obviously help reduce or eliminate straining and irritation.

A Natural Reducing Aid

There are many appetite suppressants on the market that cannot do much more for the individual wanting to lose weight than water can do. By drinking six to eight glasses of water daily, the weight-conscious individual gains a full feeling that helps combat the desire for food. Here, I want to emphasize that I am not advocating that water be used as a replacement for the regular meals of the day. Instead, it can be used at meals to forestall the desire for second and third helpings. Also, it can be used between meals to curb snacking on sweets, donuts, and other junk food. In the face of all of the diet books and articles, the use of plain water as a weight-reducing aid seems too simple. The trend in weight reduction is to the complicated, with charts, menus, and regimes. But the use of water as an appetite suppressant can and does work. Combine it with the COSS method mentioned in another chapter, and you have a simple and inexpensive weight-reduction routine.

In the event the individual on a weight-reducing regime finds chemically treated tap water not to his or her liking, there are many spring waters available to be used as substitutes.

An Excellent Diuretic

An additional benefit for the overweight individual is that water helps with a high-blood pressure problem. The increased intake of water produces a diuretic effect. Water is an excellent diuretic and helps rid the body of sodium, helping relieve hypertension. To compensate for the accompanying loss of potassium, the individual should increase the intake of fruits and vegetables that are high in potassium.

In addition, straining to effect a bowel movement can be harmful to the patient with a heart problem. By helping soften stools, water helps the heart patient avoid straining at the time of the bowel movement.

An Important Lubricant

Water is a lubricant, even though it's not oily or greasy. It helps in the lubrication of joints and the movement of the organs in the abdominal cavity.

An Aid to Electrolytic Balance

When carbohydrates are broken down, they form such acids as lactic acid. Ordinarily, this is broken down further to give carbon dioxide and water. Fats are normally split into fatty acids and glycerol. If everything is normal, further reduction occurs to produce carbon dioxide and water. On the other hand, most fruits and vegetables are basic in reaction.

Thus, in coping with these chemical reactions, the body needs water to help in the constant adjustment of the electrolyte balance in cells and in the blood.

The All-Around Health Booster

To have a well-rounded and balanced diet, be sure to obtain an adequate intake of water as has been outlined here. By doing so you will be aiding the digestion of foods, the transport and distribution of nutrients, the maintenance of the important electrolytic balance of bodily fluids and blood, and the elimination of waste products.

Dr. Daro's Nutritional Solutions to Medical Problems

Chapter 7

Nutrition and Medical Problems

In spite of the fact that we have more trained medical professionals, improved diagnostic procedures, more effective drugs, and better medical facilities, we have more people who are ill and require medical attention. Why is this?

While stress, air pollution, alcohol, tobacco, street drugs, breakdown in moral values, water supplies, nuclear radiation, and many other factors are indicted as causes of medical problems, my experience has led me to believe that faulty nutrition is one of the underlying causes. I also believe that nutritional science is the wave of the future in medial practice. I am encouraged to see that renowned educators are proposing changes that will produce medical professionals oriented toward prevention. Derek C. Bok, president of Harvard University, recently urged medical school reforms among which was the recommendation that faculties offer better instruction in preventive medicine. It was pointed out that half of all illness in the United States could be avoided through voluntary adjustments in lifestyle. In my medical practice experience, a key adjustment in "lifestyle" is what we decide to put inside of the only body we will ever have.

Poor Nutrition Is Everywhere

While poor nutrition is more outwardly apparent in less-developed countries, it still exerts a powerful effect on the physical and mental energy of our country's population. In one study it was estimated that as many as 40 million people in the United States, for example, have a nutritional lack of some kind. It was found that 25 percent of the study group had an iron deficiency, along with unacceptable levels of vitamin C, protein, riboflavin, folic acid, and thiamine.

Good Nutrition—First Step in Conquering Overweight

While we may not have the emaciated by our roadsides, we have another obvious example of poor nutrition among us and that is the overweight individual. Consuming calories beyond physical needs is the simplest way of defining what causes obesity. In the United States, estimates range from 20 to 30 percent of the population as having an excess weight problem. What makes this fact disturbing is that the obese have a greater chance of developing cardiovascular disease, diabetes, digestive tract diseases, malignancies, and cerebral accidents.

Sound nutritional planning will produce a more attractive and slimmed-down you. Even more important is that we will steer you away from the more catastrophic problems mentioned in the preceding paragraph.

Nutrition and Mental Health

In the treatment of mental disease, good results are being obtained using a nutritional approach. A zinc-manganese supplement has been used to treat schizophrenia. Investigators at the New Jersey Neuropsychiatric Institute observed that high copper levels are often associated with psychiatric symptoms and that copper is excreted poorly by many suffering schizophrenia. Zinc is a copper antagonist and aids in copper excretion.

Manic-depressive states are being treated using a nutritional approach. Lithium carbonate has been found to calm the manic phase and, simultaneously, diminish the depressive state as well. In a three-year study that compared El Paso and Dallas, it was found that Dallas experienced three times as many admissions for personality disorders. It was further found that

El Paso has 130 micrograms of lithium per liter of drinking water while Dallas has no lithium in its water.

How the overall diet influences behavior patterns has been demonstrated in animal studies. In one such study, a control group of 20 rats were housed together in a large cage and provided with a diet containing key nutrients. This group thrived, developed, and adjusted well to each other. Another group of twenty rats was given similar quarters but was furnished a diet consisting of low-nutrient, high-calorie foods. Rats in this group developed hair that was lusterless, exhibited irritability, and bit each other. In a short time, they became cannibalistic and killed three of their own kind. To complete the experiment, it was necessary to separate the animals in individual cages.

Is there a relationship between experiments such as these and the mental health of humans? Is it possible that part of the problems afflicting society—more divorces, increased juvenile delinquency, higher crime rate—might have roots in the nutritional deterioration of our diets? In my opinion a sufficient amount of research and clinical work has been done to say that the answer is yes.

I don't think that you and I have to understand all of the activities going on in the operation of the brain and nervous system to know instinctively that nutrients we supply or skip can probably affect their performance. If alcohol, for example, can dim or put out the lights in our brains, so to speak, there should be nutritional substances with positive, or at least helpful, effects.

I review some of my findings and experiences in applying nutrients to improved mental functioning in the chapter, "Mental Health."

Nutrition for Cardiovascular Health

In the same way, the proper functioning of the cardiovascular system can be related to the correct combination of trace elements in the diet. One study showed that persons living in a particular region of Georgia had 50 percent fewer heart attacks and strokes than a similar group living in another part of the state.

The evidence that was available pointed to the fact that the only difference was a higher exposure to trace elements in food and water of the "protected" group. An analysis of the soil showed higher concentrations of aluminum, barium, calcium, chromium, copper, iron, potassium, magnesium, manganese, niobium, phosphorus, titanium, and vanadium.

Other researchers have noted that low magnesium has been incriminated for causing atherosclerosis through two different mechanisms that involve raising cholesterol levels in the blood and encouraging calcification of the vascular walls. In related research, it was shown that there was an association between estrogen therapy and an increased tendency for blood clotting to occur. This was corrected by oral magnesium therapy.

The important role of trace elements is to catalyze the synthesis of cellular enzymes that, in turn, direct and accelerate the chemical reactions vital to cellular processes of growth, repair, and maintenance.

Good Nutrition—Help for Many Medical Problems

Many other medical problems can be helped through good nutritional practices. By helping patients modify their diets, I have had good results with a variety of complaints and illnesses, such as cardiovascular, skin, cyst, tension, and insomnia problems. In the following chapters of this book, I illustrate specific conditions that have been helped. Yet, let me emphasize that sound eating plans and supplementation should not be viewed as one-time shots. I want you to come away from reading this book with the idea that diet improvement with the inclusion of key vitamins and minerals is a plan for all phases of your life. Nutritional therapy can be modified to meet special conditions but I want you to set in place the framework to help you live a better total life.

Chapter 8

Mental Health

In the chapter, "Nutrition and Medical Problems," I suggested that a relationship exists between nutrition and the functioning of the nervous system. I mentioned that if a substance like alcohol can shut down or inhibit mental performance, perhaps there are nutrients that can do just the opposite.

The effect of nutrients on mental health and performance is one of the newest and most exciting areas of investigation and progress in health care. Later in this chapter I'll mention the results I have had from taking two amino acids. Until now, the brain, nervous system, and human behavior have largely been the domain of psychiatrists and psychologists. Medical researchers, however, have learned more about the biochemistry of the transmission of nerve impulses and the chemicals manufactured by the brain to demonstrate that behavior modification and improved mental performance are possible through nutritional means. If we can improve, for example, the performance of the cardiovascular system through diet modification, then it's logical to assume that comparable nutritional changes might just help the way the brain and nervous system function.

Whole-Body Nutrition Comes First

To start with, good mental performance and health depend on good, whole-body functioning. What is nutritionally important, generally, for the cardiovascular, digestive, and skeletal systems will have a positive effect on the brain and central nervous system. Above and beyond that, research and clinical study have shown that certain nutrients have a special role in promoting proper functioning of the nervous system. Just as special chemicals, enzymes, and hormones are manufactured by various tissues and organs elsewhere in the body, so do the brain and central nervous system manufacture and use unique chemicals for their functioning. In both cases the building blocks for the manufacture of the chemicals come from the food we eat.

Investigators have connected certain mental health problems to nutritional deficiencies. The table below lists some of these relationships. The right-hand column is headed, "Mental Health Problems." I wish to emphasize that the nutritional deficiencies given affect other body systems as well, as the symptoms given may be just part of the total problem. In addition, the table should not be used as a therapeutic guide for solving the symptoms or problems listed. Only in consultation with a nutritionally-knowledgeable physician should a course of therapy be outlined.

Nutrient Deficiency	Mental Health Problem
vitamin B-1 (thiamine)	depression, memory loss, noise sensitivity
vitamin B-2 (riboflavin)	depression
niacinamide	depression, nervousness, irritability
vitamin B-6 (pyridoxine)	irritability, convulsions, tension
vitamin B-12 (cobalamin)	emotional disorders including insanity, memory loss, difficulty in concentration
biotin	lassitude
calcium	insomnia, nervousness, apathy
magnesium	twitching, tremors, confusion, disorientation
potassium	depression (also necessary for nerve activity)
vitamin C (ascorbic acid)	diminished mental alertness
vitamin D	increase in nervous system irritability caused by low blood calcium
vitamin E	nervous disorders
sodium chloride	lessening of mental acuity

As the preceding list of nutrients suggests (and it is an incomplete one), you and I need to construct our diets from a variety of food sources to obtain the nutrients necessary for a properly functioning brain and nervous sytem. It is apparent that we need virtually the whole spectrum of vitamins and minerals. Next, to cover up any sins of omission in our eating programs, it seems wise to supplement with a vitamin-mineral formulation. Then, if there are specific problems that might need specific nutrient materials, we can embark on a program with nutritional guidance to treat or help the nervous system symptom.

My Nutritional Therapy for Mental Health Problems

In my practice, as with many physicians, I have patients with nervous system problems, such as hyperexcitability, nervousness, memory loss, signs of early senility, depression, apathy, and substandard mental performance. I, of course, will do physical examinations and have diagnostic tests run to determine if any serious pathologies or neurological problems are involved. If the results are negative, I review the diet of the patients to learn if there are deficiencies that can be related to the symptoms.

The Highly Excitable Patient

A typical patient was the attractive mother of two teenagers, 42 years of age, who was recently divorced after 18 years of marriage. When she came in, she was obviously highly agitated and continuously twisted a handkerchief in her hands. She immediately requested a prescription for tranquilizers. I stopped prescribing tranquilizers long ago and advised her of this. I remembered the last time I saw her some years back, when she was a calm and delightful woman. She complained that the divorce, increased responsibilities in her job, and trying to be a single parent had just ganged up on her. She said that she was snapping at her children more and that she was having a difficult time controlling her emotions at work when the assignments piled up.

After the physical examination and tests turned up nothing out of the ordinary, I explained that any real long-term improvement and ability to cope with the new stresses in her life would not come from tranquilizers. I said that there was a good possibility that diet modification might help. As I delved into her diet, I learned that she had virtually stopped eating breakfast at home. Instead, she stopped before work for a cup of coffee and a donut. Then, throughout the morning, she had more coffee and sometimes a candy bar. Lunch consisted of a salad. Her only real meal was dinner prepared by her teenage daughter. Instead of more and better nutrient intake to meet a high-stress situation, she was getting less and depleting whatever reserves her body had. She was getting very few B vitamins, not much calcium for its calming effect, and her protein component was way down.

What was needed was a little time management to permit her to make breakfast at home, and instruction to guide her to a more diverse selection of foods for her lunches. She agreed to give herself more time in the mornings and to start with fresh fruit or juices, soft or poached eggs alternating with whole grain cereals, and milk. To lessen her craving for a midmorning candy bar, I suggested that maybe a small bag of soybeans or a piece of fruit might help her through. For her lunches, I directed her attention to more protein choices, such as tuna, lean beef, or chicken. Even a peanut butter sandwich brought from home was suggested as an alternative. The dinners were generally satisfactory with the exception that I wanted her to include a wider variety of vegetables in her salads—more carrots, tomatoes, broccoli, etc., instead of just lettuce. I prescribed a vitamin-mineral formulation, additional vitamin C because I thought her immune system needed to build up, a vitamin B stress formulation, and a chelated calcium-magnesium supplement for its calmative effect.

The patient returned after a month and reported that she had noted an improvement after three weeks on the program. She said that she was having trouble getting to sleep and I prescribed tryptophan, one of the essential amino acids. On her next visit, she said that she was now able to sleep soundly and that she was "in control of the events" in her life. She certainly presented a calm appearance, as she sat opposite me in my office with none of the previous handkerchief twisting and ringing around her hands.

By far, the largest number of patients whom I have treated for nervousness, tension, insomnia, and depression have invariably been following the same eating pattern of sweet rolls, donuts, coffee, soft drinks, snack foods, and other empty or nearly empty-calorie foods substituting for meat, eggs, cheese, fruit, vegetables, and whole grain breads and cereals. And, when we do convince the patients to trade in the old diets for new, nutritionally sound eating patterns, we have yet to have a patient disappointed with the results.

The Older, Mentally Confused Patient

At another end of the mental health spectrum was the 75-year-old mother of a patient. The patient told me that her mother had been living with her for the past two years since the death of her father. While the first year and a half had been uneventful, the next six months had seen her mother becoming more forgetful and even confused about operating appliances like the television, toaster, and even the stove; she was also eating less. I asked her to take her mother to the hospital for a thorough diagnostic work-up. Mental deterioration and senility are certainly not unusual at this age. Obviously, not all such cases can be easily treated through nutritional means.

The results of the tests showed no major problems, except an obvious loss of weight from previous levels. When the two came in together, it was apparent that the mother was suffering from depression. She said that she had no complaints and that her daughter was making a big fuss over nothing.

Since she had been a prolific cook in earlier years, the daughter and I devised a strategy to let the mother plan the meals for the family on alternate days. As she got involved in meal planning and preparation, she started to eat more and her spirits were lifted.

In addition, in cases of this kind, I have had good results with lecithin. The reason for this approach is that impaired brain functioning can be related to the build-up of deposits of cholesterol in the blood vessels of the brain. Lecithin helps unclog any such deposits, and the nourishment of brain cells is improved. At the same time, we are helping break up any cholesterol deposits in the blood supply of the heart. In this manner we contribute to the more efficient pumping action of the heart in sending blood to the brain and throughout the body. Lecithin is available in the form of granules and I told the daughter to sprinkle it on whatever foods the mother might be eating. In addition, since lecithin is manufactured by the body, I recommended foods high in choline, which is the building block for lecithin. Choline is also involved in the production of acetylcholine which is a chemical transmitter of nerve impulses. Food sources of choline include liver, kidneys, fish, egg yolk, beans, wheat germ, peanuts, and yeast.

I also prescribed a nonessential amino acid, glutamine, which is converted by the body into a useful brain fuel and has been used to improve functioning of the brain. This, with a vitamin B complex and a vitamin-mineral formulation, was the nutritional therapy provided. Regarding the diet, the mother had always instinctively eaten well without any coaching.

I did not hear from the daughter for a while. Three months later she came in for a check-up and reported how pleased she was with her mother's progress. The mother was more alert and no longer displayed the confusion and depression of her former state. She ate well and had regained most of the weight previously lost.

The Mentally Retarded Patient

Recently I treated a young, 14-year-old mentally retarded boy using a combination of amino acids with very promising results. I became aware of the youngster and his problems while visiting a friend where the boy's mother works. Knowing that I was a physician, she talked to me about his condition and the many clinics and physicians she had examine him. She also told me that caring for the boy, as many parents of retarded children will testify, can be emotionally draining, tiring, and stressful. She recited some of his problems, including frequent crying episodes, strong attachment to her, depression, and poor performance in the school he attends.

I saw the boy subsequently and asked his mother if she would be willing to try something with him involving amino acids. She agreed quite readily and I could understand that she was hopeful for some help and improvement in his condition. I recommended glutamine because it has been reported to improve the intelligence of mentally retarded children. Next, I said he should take tyrosine because it has an effect in controlling anxiety and depression. Finally, I prescribed tryptophan. Tryptophan is used by the body to make serotonin, which affects emotional states, promotes a calm attitude, and is needed for sleep.

The results after four to six weeks of treatment and as reported to me by the mother have been almost astonishing. Here's what she has told me has occurred in his behavior:

1. He is more mature, less childish, and not clinging to his mother like before.
2. Crying episodes have decreased in frequency.
3. His father is in the real estate business and the boy looks for, and identifies news items pertaining to the field, clips them out, and gives them to his father.
4. There is less of a problem now taking him shopping. Previously, he did not want to go and would refuse to enter shops and stores.
5. He likes school now. His teacher says that his math skills have improved, his memory span is greater, and he doesn't make noise in the classroom anymore. He also writes better and, for the first time, he is attending summer school.
6. He also:
   a. sleeps better.
   b. takes the amino acids and vitamins by himself without being told.
   c. is easier to live with.

I want to caution that readers with mentally retarded children should not immediately go out and try this same therapeutic method with their offspring. Find a nutrition-oriented physician, ask him about amino acids as a possible treatment, and discuss how or if they might benefit your loved one.

Other Natural Ways to Boost Your Brain Power

In addition to B vitamins, calcium, magnesium, and lecithin contributing to brain and nervous system performance, the amino acids are drawing interest.

Glutamic Acid/Glutamine. Some investigators suggest that glutamic acid, a nonessential amino acid, can improve intelligence. A problem with glutamic acid as a nutrient is that only a limited amount can cross the protective blood barrier of the brain. However, a chemical relation, L-glutamine, can readily cross the barrier and be converted into glutamic acid. Investigators have used glutamine with apparent positive results in cases of senility, schizophrenia, mental retardation, and petit mal epilepsy. Its use has also been stated to curb the use of alcohol and sweets.

Tryptophan. This is an essential amino acid that is converted inside the brain into serotonin. Serotonin controls emotions and perception of pain, elevates moods of depression, produces a calm attitude, and promotes sleep. It is also reported that migraine sufferers have lower levels of serotonin than the normal population. Tryptophan is reported to be more effective when taken with vitamin B-6 (pyridoxine) and vitamin C, both of which are necessary for its metabolism. For the past few months I have been taking tryptophan and have found it very useful as a sleep-inducing agent. Natural sources of tryptophan include poultry, lean meats, nuts, and milk.

Phenylalanine. This is also an essential amino acid and is one of the few amino acids readily converted into basic brain compounds that control mood. It is the raw material used by the brain to produce compounds that transmit nerve impulses. Norepinephrine is one of these along with adrenalin and dopamine. These compounds formed within the brain are responsible for an elevated and positive mood, alertness, and ambition. Phenylalanine is particularly high in nonfat dried milk; other sources include eggs, lean meat, poultry, and fish.

I have been taking phenylalanine for its mood-elevating effect and can report satisfactory results from this therapy.

Tyrosine. This is a nonessential amino acid that is manufactured from phenylalanine. Because of this relationship, it is involved in the production of norepinephrine. Tyrosine also has a mood-elevating effect and in one research study, two patients with long-standing depressions experienced improvement after conventional drug therapy proved ineffective.

Common Food Sources of Powerful Brain Boosters

Amino acids are derived from protein sources. In general, proteins of animal origin, e.g., milk, eggs, meat, poultry, fish, along with soybean protein, have the highest biologic value. This is a value assigned on the basis of the quantity and quality of the amino acid composition. Whole eggs rank first in this system. In the second group are cereals, nuts, and legumes. Cereal grain proteins are low in lysine, which promotes bone growth, as is corn protein in tryptophan. However, when cereals are used as mixtures with other proteins, particularly milk, eggs, or meat, the overall combination is excellent in amino acid content. Vegetables are incomplete sources of amino acids and fruits supply even less.

Vegetarians, in particular, have to be careful in planning their meals in order to obtain the full complement of essential amino acids. As suggested in the preceding paragraph, combining different foods is necessary to come up with the required amounts of the amino acids.

For readers interested in learning more about the amino acid content of foods, you may want to consult nutritional text books or, "Composition of Foods," U.S. Department of Agriculture, Human Nutritive Service, Agricultural Handbooks 8-1 through 8-12, which are available through the Superintendent of Documents, U.S. Government Printing Office, Washington, D.C. 20402.

The preceding discussion reinforces the idea that you and I need a well-balanced diet to assure ourselves of the nutritional elements necessary for brain and nerve power. Each of us, because of individual biologic makeup, might need certain nutritional elements more than others. As I mentioned I am taking tryptophan to help induce sleep and phenylalanine for its mood-elevating qualities. For your own particular symptoms and needs, I strongly recommend that you consult with a nutritionally expert physician.

Chapter 9

Cancer

The following are a few thoughts, observations, and experiences relating to cancer, nutrition, and the immune system of the body.

Just as there are many types of bacteria and viruses that are responsible for infections in the body, so there are many cancer-causing agents and phenomena. Some of the factors having the potential for causing cancer are naturally occurring phenomena with which we come into contact on almost a daily basis. For example, sunlight can be potentially harmful. Solar energy in the form of rays reaching the earth is at once lethal and beneficial, depending on the length of exposure. Sunlight helps promote the production of vitamin D in the body. Overexposure to the rays of the sun, however, has been identified as a potentially causative factor of skin cancer. A higher incidence of skin cancer is documented among people living in sunny climates. However, not all people who subject themselves to an excess of sunlight automatically develop skin cancer. Some people will develop skin cancer, some will not.

There are other factors in our environment that are potentially hazardous and cancer causing. These factors are the price we pay for our advancing industrialization and technological progress. They include the airborne pollutants, fumes, dusts, mists, chemicals, and other emissions from auto exhausts, steel mills, chemical plants, nuclear plants, office and home heating systems, incinerators, waste disposal sites, airplanes, trucks, and locomotives. There is also the battle being waged to clean up our lakes, streams, and rivers from the ravages of chemicals and other waste products being dumped into them. Water supplies are, thus, another potential source of cancer-causing factors. The food that we eat has been suspected at times because of coloring, preservatives, artificial sweetening, and synthetic flavoring agents. Sodium nitrite, which has been used extensively in meat products such as bacon and hotdogs, has been cited as carcinogenic. There is a continuing scientific battle being waged on the suspected carcinogenicity of the artificial sweetener, saccharin.

The workplace is another source of potential cancer-causing factors. The worker may not only be exposed to airborne fumes and dusts, but also to direct contact with liquids, powders, and solid materials. High heat may be part of the hazards in the work environment.

Stress is another factor cited as cancer causing. The stress may not only be the factory but also the office, laboratory, or executive suite. It may be a factor in the home environment, also.

Some people exposed to these factors and phenomena develop cancer and others do not.

Why?

I believe part of the answer lies with the body's immune system. And, the efficiency of the body's immune system is undoubtedly associated with hereditary factors.

The tuberculosis bacillus causes tuberculosis and pneumococcus bacteria bring on pneumonia. Viruses cause diseases like small pox, chicken pox, mumps, and infantile paralysis. From some of these bacterial and viral diseases, researchers have been successful in developing vaccines that fight the infections and confer immunity. They work by stimulating the body's own immune system to develop antibodies that combat and destroy the invading virus or bacteria.

The importance of the immune system is illustrated by what has been observed of patients undergoing organ transplant surgery. In this type of surgery, it is the practice for the immune system to be suppressed by the use of cortisone to counteract rejection of the organ transplant. It was discovered that a number of these patients developed cancer. This occurrence called attention to the importance of the immune system in fighting cancer. And, currently, many groups direct their attention in the fight against cancer by seeking to develop cancer vaccines or otherwise stimulate the activity of the body's own defensive mechanism—the immune system.

Thus, the immune system plays a key role in preventing infections and in combating foreign invaders—in the example cited, it turns out to be an organ transplant. This phenomenon also points up the factor of biological individuality. While it is true that the transplant is coming from another human being, the body has a way of recognizing that the tissue is different in makeup and considers the transplanted organ a foreign invader.

It stands to reason that in keeping with the theory of biological individuality, all immune systems will not be in a similar state of readiness to repel the foreign, destructive factor; whatever its purpose. In addition to whatever hereditary characteristics we possess individually, I believe that the functioning of the immune system is related to a soundly conceived nutritional program. Our immune systems in each of our bodies are in different states of readiness to repel attack by disease. This helps explain why some heavy smokers develop cancer and others do not and, generally, why exposure to other carcinogenic materials or factors produces dissimilar effects in different bodies.

Helping the Immune System through Nutrition

In my view, the optimum functioning of the immune system is related to maintaining an optimal level of nutritional intake. Furnishing the body with all of the vitamins, minerals, amino acids, and high-quality protein through a balanced diet and by supplementation is the basic starting point for an optimally functioning immune system. In addition, I believe that extra quantities of vitamins A and C, and the mineral selenium, are necessary. These particular nutrient materials have demonstrated special effectiveness in combating infection.

Obesity and Diabetes—Cancer Connection?

One of my clinical observations is that obesity and diabetes seem prevalent in many patients who develop cancer of the breast or cancer of the endometrium or inner lining of the uterus.

When I was performing surgery and doing hysterectomies for endometrial cancer following irradiation, I noted that a high percentage of the patients were obese. Overall, in my experience, I can say that I found a larger percentage of obese patients having surgery for breast cancer.

Influence of Vitamin A on Cancer

In one experiment two groups of rats were given cortisone to lower the white blood cell count that, as previously mentioned, suppresses the immune system. One group of rats, however, was also given vitamin A. The finding was that the group receiving cortisone but no vitamin A experienced a significant lowering of the white blood cell count. The other group receiving the supplemental vitamin A along with the cortisone had little or no lowering of the white blood cell count.

Vitamin C and Cancer

Dr. Linus Pauling has conducted and is sponsoring research in the use of megadoses of vitamin C in treating cancer. The results seem to show a prolongation of life.

Personal Experiences with Nutrition and Cancer

I have always made it a practice when I have operated on a patient with cancer to encourage a sound nutritional program. This has included vitamins A and C and a broad-spectrum vitamin and mineral formulation.

One of my patients was a female, 50 years of age, who was operated on for cancer of the ovaries. We discovered that the cancer had spread throughout the abdomen and involved the liver. The prognosis was not optimistic because of the massive involvement of the other organs. Nevertheless, irradiation and chemotherapy were prescribed. In addition, I urged her to eat well and to never miss a meal. Also, if her appetite was reduced because of the treatment she was receiving, I suggested that she eat four to six smaller meals daily. I prescribed a complete supplementation program including a vitamin-mineral combination preparation, six grams of vitamin C, and 30,000 units of vitamin A each day. I was encouraged that the patient lived some three years following the surgery and attribute this survival period to the assistance she obtained from the nutritional program.

Dietary Guidelines from the National Academy of Sciences' Committee on Diet, Nutrition, and Cancer

The Committee on Diet, Nutrition, and Cancer of the National Academy of Sciences' National Research Council evaluated four decades of scientific studies and evidence concerning cancer and its relationship to certain dietary patterns and individual dietary components. While concluding that the evidence pointed to a direct correlation between diet and various types of cancers, the study group stepped back from attempting to say to what degree diet might influence the onset of cancer. They went on to say that the case for dietary influences on human cancers was reinforced by observing that similar dietary patterns and components of food also affected the incidence of certain cancers in animals.

The study points out that because diets vary so widely in populations and many factors can influence the development of chronic diseases besides diet, it is not likely that a precise diet can be formulated that will protect everyone against all forms of cancer. Nevertheless, the Committee on Diet, Nutrition, and Cancer determined that the evidence was sufficient to make certain interim dietary reocmmenations.

Intake of Fat. Because the occurrence of cancer appears to be linked with fat intake, the amount of calories coming from fats in the diet should be cut to 30 percent. The correlation between fat intake seem to be strongest for cancers of the breast, colon, and prostate. The recommendation, then, is to eat lean cuts of beef, fish, and chicken, and to eliminate or reduce intake of butter, cream, and foods or meals prepared in saturated oils and greases—french fries, donuts, snack foods, pies, and cakes.

Importance of Fruits, Vegetables, and Whole-Grain Cereals. It is important to include fruits, vegetables, and whole-grain cereal products in the daily diet, especially citrus fruits, and carotene-rich and cabbage family vegetables. Carotene, also known as provitamin A, is transformed by the body into vitamin A. Carotene-rich foods include dark green and deep yellow vegetables like carrots, sweet potatoes, and members of the cruiciferae family, such as cabbage, cauliflower, Brussels sprouts and broccoli. The family includes mustards, watercress, kale, collards, turnips, kohlrabi, rutabagas, and radishes.

Studies of the incidence of cancer in Norway, Japan, Hawaii, and the continental United States found a lower risk of cancer of the stomach among individuals who ate large quantities of vegetables. For example, one particular study found less stomach cancer in people who traditionally eat raw vegetables, including cole slaw and red cabbage than among people who do not consume as much of these vegetables.

Comparing cases of colon and rectal cancer among hospital patients with other people in the community, it has been shown that there is less cancer of the colon among those eating cabbage and similar high-fiber foods. Studies in such geographically distant places as Minnesota, Japan, and upstate New York similarly demonstrated that there was a lessened risk of developing colon cancer when there was frequent consumption of raw broccoli, cabbage, and Brussels sprouts, as well as other vegetables.

Citrus fruits, of course, provide large amounts of vitamin C and, also, are high in fiber content when eaten raw. Oranges and grapefruit are the most readily available citrus fruits.

The whole grain cereals are those that have a high content of whole wheat, oats, and bran. In the event that the cereal you are using does not contain the grain in its raw or natural state, an addition of two or three tablespoons of raw wheat germ is an excellent way to upgrade the cereal.

Reduce or Eliminate Cured, Smoked, and Pickled Foods. Researchers have found a correlation between the intake of cured, smoked, and pickled foods and esophageal cancer in China, and a higher incidence of stomach cancer in Japan, U.S.S.R., Iceland, Hungary, and the United States. In a number of these cases, there is an apprent correlation between the consumption of smoked and pickled fish and stomach cancer. It is interesting that certain high-risk counties exist in Wisconsin, Minnesota, and Michigan where eating habits are apparently transplanted from a Scandinavian country like Norway.

The recommendation seems to be quite clear in this shaping of a diet to avoid and minimize cancer risk—foods like smoked herring and other fish, bacons, hams, and other related products are to be eaten negligibly, if at all.

Stay Away from Alcohol. Alcohol is the most powerful beverage in the diet that has been identified as causing cancer in humans, especially if consumed in conjunction with cigarette smoking. The effects of alcohol do not appear to be related to the 1500 odd compounds present in alcoholic drinks but on the ethyl alcohol itself. Some research people believe that ethyl alcohol is a promoter by itself. Other researchers regard it as a solvent that increases the local absorption of cancer-causing substances in the esophagus.

Cancer and Weight. Workers in the field agree that overeating may be linked to cancer promotion in animals and probably in humans. With the possible exception of cancer of the thyroid as related to an iodine deficiency and cancer of the hypopharynx as related to an iron deficiency, no human cancer has been attributed solely to a dietary deficiency. There are reports, however, that show that undernutrition in animals may actually inhibit spontaneous and experimental cancer at different sites in the animals. The relationship between undernutrition and a decreased cancer risk seems to be one of the most agreed-upon observations in the field of diet and nutrition.

I think it is important for you to maintain an ideal body weight to avoid obesity, for in the process you reduce the probability of other chronic disorders.

It is also important in following these guidelines that you don't go overboard in consuming extra large quantities of any one of the foods mentioned. There is still an extraordinary amount of research that needs to be done in finding links between diet and cancer. While there seems to be no disagreement among investigators concerning the role that diet plays in human cancers, there is a range of opinion as to the importance of individual factors in the diet. Thus, the sensible reader interested in health maintenance and disease prevention will stay alert to new findings as they are announced by recognized research institutions and make adjustments in his or her diet under the guidance of a medical practitioner with nutritional experience.

Important Cancer-Fighting Foods

Because I believe in the importance of vitamins A and C and the mineral, selenium, in cancer prevention, important sources of these nutritional factors are listed in the following tables.*

		Vitamin A International Units	Vitamin C Milligrams
Fruits			
apricots, raw	3 apricots	2,890	4
apricots, dried, uncooked	1 cup	14,170	16
apricots, canned in heavy syrup	1 cup	4,490	10
avocados, raw	1 avocado	630	30
cantaloupe, raw, orange flesh	½ melon	9,240	90
cherries, tart, red, canned, water pack	1 cup	1,660	12
cherries, sweet, raw	10 cherries	70	7
grapefruit, raw, pink/red	½ grapefruit	540	44
grapefruit juice, fresh, red flesh	1 cup	1,080	93
oranges, raw	1 orange	260	66
orange juice, fresh	1 cup	500	124
orange juice, frozen, diluted	1 cup	540	120
papayas, raw	1 cup	2,450	78
peaches, raw, yellow flesh	1 peach	1,330	7
prunes, cooked, unsweetened	1 cup	1,590	2
strawberries, raw	1 cup	90	88
tangerines, raw	1 tangerine	360	27
watermelon, raw, 4 × 6-inch wedge	1 wedge	2,510	30

*Information is derived from Home and Garden Bulletin No. 72, "Nutritive Value of Foods," revised April 1981 and published by U.S. Dept. of Agriculture.

Vegetables		Vitamin A International Units	Vitamin C Milligrams
asparagus, green, raw, cuts and tips	1 cup	1,310	38
beans, snap, green, cooked & drained	1 cup	680	15
beet greens, cooked & drained	1 cup	7,400	22
broccoli, stalk, cooked, & drained	1 cup	4,500	162
brussels sprouts, cooked & drained	1 cup	810	135
cabbage, raw, shredded	1 cup	90	33
carrots, raw, whole	1 carrot	7,930	6
carrots, cooked & drained	1 cup	16,280	9
collards, cooked & drained	1 cup	14,820	144
dandelion greens, cooked & drained	1 cup	12,290	19
kale, cooked & drained	1 cup	9,130	102
lettuce, raw	1 wedge	450	8
mustard greens, cooked & drained	1 cup	8,120	67
peas, green, cooked & drained, canned	1 cup	1,170	14
potatoes, baked	1 potato	trace	31
pumpkin, canned	1 cup	15,680	12
spinach, raw	1 cup	4,460	28
spinach, cooked & drained	1 cup	14,580	50
squash, winter, baked, mashed	1 cup	8,610	27
sweet potatoes, baked in skin	1 potato	9,230	25
sweet potatoes, canned solid pack	1 cup	19,890	36
tomatoes, raw	1 tomato	1,110	28
turnip greens, cooked & drained	1 cup	8,270	68

Selenium

As is mentioned in the chapter on selenium, the U.S. has relatively selenium-poor soil. How much selenium we obtain is dependent on the region of the country where we live. Anyone wishing to be sure of obtaining at least a maintenance amount of selenium should eat from as wide a variety as possible of various foods. Good selenium foods are seafood, whole grains, organ meats, garlic, onion, and yeast. Many multivitamin and mineral formulations are now including selenium. While there is no recommended daily allowance, the Food and Nutrition Board has suggested a dietary intake of 50 to 200 micrograms of selenium per day.

Chapter 10

Multiple Sclerosis

Multiple sclerosis is a neurological disease that results in the progressive destruction of the myelin, or sheath covering the message-carrying nerve fibers in the brain and spinal cord. The process is called demyelination, and where the myelin is destroyed, it is replaced by plaques of hardened tissue that interfere with the transmission of nerve impulses. Approximately two-thirds of the cases occur between the ages of 20 and 40. It is estimated that 500,000 people in the U.S. have multiple sclerosis.

How and why multiple sclerosis strikes is not well understood. There are a number of conditions that can destroy myelin, including but not limited to viral infection, antibodies, and carbon monoxide poisoning. One line of thinking, for example, is that a virus infection occurs early in life and that the virus is in a latent state before conditions are right for it to carry out its destructive action.

Another view is that the body's process of manufacturing myelin may not progress properly due to malnourishment of the fetus, where it starts to occur around the fifth month, and the early developmental years of the child. This theory provides a very strong argument for the pregnant woman to follow sound nutritional practices to provide the fetus with a chance for proper development and subsequent healthy growth after birth. It is an intriguing thought, isn't it, that women before, during, and after pregnancies can practice, in its truest sense, preventive medicine by following good nutrition. Who knows how much of the nation's health bill they might save through reducing the amount of treatment medicine that is practiced?

Symptoms of Multiple Sclerosis

The symptoms of multiple sclerosis are varied and the degree of severity depends on where the demyelination has occurred in the central nervous system and how far it has progressed. The symptoms include weakness of arms and legs, unsteady walk, loss of sensation or numbness to touch, pain or high temperature, poorly articulated speech, visual disturbance, urinary and bowel problems, loss of balance, depression, tremor, irritability, and fatigue.

Nutritional Therapy for MS

A number of nutritional approaches have been proposed in treating multiple sclerosis. One of these is a balanced, gluten-free diet. This means that foods containing wheat and rye are excluded.

Another diet combines a low-fat with a gluten-free diet, and adds supplements of vitamins and minerals. The proponent of this diet, Roger MacDougall, held that the combination was responsible for the almost complete disappearance of his symptoms of multiple sclerosis.

Dr. Roy L. Swank, Professor Emeritus of the Department of Neurology, University of Oregon Medical School, has advocated a diet low in saturated fatty acids, as might be derived from animal fat, processed (hydrogenated) vegetable oils, and coconut and palm oil. He defines these products as solid or hard at refrigerator temperatures. Instead of these products, he favors those substances containing mainly unsaturated fatty acids found in vegetable and fish oils. These are liquid at refrigerator temperatures.

Very briefly, the diet suggests that no more than three teaspoons (15 grams) of fat be consumed daily as obtained from meat, poultry, liver, and eggs. Fat-containing red meats are limited to only two days per week. On the other hand, the diet recommends no less than four teaspoons (20 grams) of oil be included in the diet as obtained from fish, nuts, and such sources of vegetable oils as safflower, corn, sunflower, soybean, cottonseed, olive, and cod liver.

It is reported that people with multiple sclerosis who follow the Swank diet live longer and, in addition, the progressive nature or worsening of the disease is said to be stemmed.

Verifying, or replicating as scientists like to say, the results obtained from these and other dietary approaches is difficult due to the unpredictable nature of multiple sclerosis. It is characterized by periods of remission and subsequent return and/or worsening of the symptoms. Because of this erratic nature of the disease, attributing positive results to a particular nutritional approach is difficult on a strictly scientific basis. We are then left with evidence that simply says that something, apparently, works.

In my dietary recommendations to patients, I am generally in agreement with the outlines of the Swank diet. I am against the use of the products of hydrogenated vegetable oils such as margarines and shortenings. These oils are treated with hydrogen to increase their stability and hardness. Hydrogenation leads to a reduction of essential fatty acids that are very important for numerous physiologic functions, including a healthy cardiovascular system promoting good blood flow.

Where I may differ with the Swank diet is that I do not restrict so severely meat and such dairy products as whole milk and various cheese products. But, in the main, the diet coincides quite closely with the diet I suggest to people for general health maintenance and improvement with emphasis on fresh fruits and vegetables, whole grain products, fish and poultry, and the avoidance of processed meat products, snack foods, pastries, and candies. Snack foods and pastries are particularly bad because of their being prepared with hydrogenated shortenings.

I believe in the viral theory as a cause for multiple sclerosis and this factor bears on the cases I have treated. At the outset, I want to point out that I have had a limited number of cases and that no one with multiple sclerosis should attempt self-treatment without the guidance of a medical doctor who is a specialist, preferably board certified, in neurology.

The first case is that of a young lady, 22 years of age, who came to me originally for the treatment of amenorrhea, or loss of her menstrual period. In taking down her medical history, I learned that she had been afflicted with multiple sclerosis for approximately two years. Her symptoms were not of the severe kind and consisted mainly of loss of position sense, slight numbness or loss of sensation in response to touch, heat, and cold, and some awkwardness in walking. She would have remissions and then a sudden return of the symptoms.

Delving into her dietary patterns, I learned that her nutritional intake was way below par. I noted that her hair lacked luster and she tended to the overweight side. I suggested that we do a hair analysis and the results showed a deficiency in magnesium, zinc, and calcium. I also learned that she smoked moderately.

I didn't like the smoking habit for its obvious deleterious effects on the cardiovascular and pulmonary systems. I pointed out to her that experiments with animals subjected to cigarette smoke produced symptoms associated with multiple sclerosis and that for any long-term improvement, she should stop as soon as possible. This was, undoubtedly, the most difficult part of the therapy for her. However, she accepted the logic of my argument and mentally stepped back and reviewed what the future might hold in store for her with respect to multiple sclerosis. It took her three months with a gradual withdrawal process but she eventually stopped smoking.

She was given my basic diet plan and especially told to eat good quality protein and load up on vegetables because of the mineral deficiencies. This was no problem for her because she found in the process that she started to lose some of her excess pounds, and this served as strong and continuing motivation. Of course, she had the rest of the diet with fruits, whole grain foods, and dairy products. We prescribed a multivitamin-mineral formulation, a little extra calcium, magnesium, and zinc, and more vitamin C. A subsequent hair analysis confirmed that the magnesium, zinc, and calcium were up to normal levels.

In keeping with my view about the connection of multiple sclerosis with a virus infection, I prescribed a dosage of six to eight grams of vitamin C. I did this because she was experiencing a return of some of the symptoms of multiple sclerosis. She reported that the therapeutic regime seemed to ameliorate the symptoms. As the symptoms subsided, I prescribed a lowered, maintenance dose in the three to four gram range, daily.

In addition to what I felt was a positive effect on the symptoms of multiple sclerosis, the nutritional regime restored her menstrual period, produced a weight loss, and gave her renewed energy and vigor.

Another case was that of an older woman who was in her 40s at the time that I saw her. She was in a wheel chair and was afflicted with multiple sclerosis when she was in her 30s. The goal here was to prevent any further deterioration of her condition. The therapeutic regime was as previously described with the extra supplementation with vitamin C. I talk to and see the lady from time to time and she reports that she has stayed with the diet plan and the extra vitamin C. As far as I can determine, there has been no slippage in her condition, which is what we had hoped for when beginning her treatment.

A third case is that of a young man who was 27 at the time that I saw him. A nurse, who was acquainted with my work in nutritional therapy, referred him to me. He had had multiple sclerosis for two years and was going through the pattern of an appearance of symptoms and then remission. He had symptoms of weakness of arms and legs, blurred vision, and tingling sensations. We followed the same treatment routine in his case and he reported back to me that when he slipped off the routine, he experienced a worsening of the symptoms.

Based on my experiences, I think that supplementation with vitamin C, as always on a foundation of a well-rounded diet, helps in multiple sclerosis. I think that multiple sclerosis is due to a viral infection and vitamin C, because of its anti-viral properties, is appropriate therapy. Elsewhere in this book, for example, I mention how I have used vitamin C to treat herpes simplex, which is a virus responsible for cold sores. I think that vitamin C is an anti-stress vitamin and, therefore, helps with the various symptoms of multiple sclerosis. In addition, vitamin C helps acidify the urine and in this way protects against bladder infections that can be another problem inflicted on the multiple sclerosis sufferer.

Again, however, I caution against self-medication. The person afflicted with multiple sclerosis should seek out a qualified neurologist. However, the National Multiple Sclerosis Society recommends sound and well-balanced diets, so that part of any treatment can begin immediately.

Chapter 11

Weight Problems

Obese...Overweight...Heavy...Fat...Stout...Plump...

Whatever word is used to describe the overweight individual, a considerable industry has grown up to help people with their excess weight problem. It could probably be called the anti-calorie industry.

Millions of words, hundreds of articles, and scores of books on weight reduction have been written and published. I think, in general, that they have served a useful purpose in directing the overweight individual to dieting, exercise, and goal setting. Where the effort to be applied is minimal such as in relying on a particular food, liquid, or product, the less satisfactory the long-term results tend to be.

In my experience with patients who have tried various plans where rigid menus are presented, shopping for the suggested food choices becomes a chore. When the food items are not available, out of season, or of poor quality from a bad crop, substitutions have to be made. This complicates the weight-reducing program. People feel guilty, get discouraged, and lose interest in what really ought to be a simple program. In addition, when eating is done away from home, the menus at restaurants and fast-food outlets make chaos out of the carefully outlined diet suggestions in the articles and books. Because of these factors, I have tried to simplify things for patients wanting to lose weight.

Special Foods

The low-calorie foods and drinks make, perhaps, the most sense in the whole panorama of weight reduction. The foods that have been developed provide an alternative to the sugar-laden and empty calorie foods that contribute to the problems of the overweight. One of the interesting developments is the emergence of canned fruits that are not steeped in the heavy and overpoweringly sweet syrups. The individual wanting to lose weight can quite easily select low-calorie frozen food entrees, soft drinks, canned fruit, and a host of other main and side dishes.

Biological Individuality

The reason for the profusion of so much information on how to lose weight is that no single method works for everyone. In my opinion, this stems from biological individuality. The causes of obesity are many. Because we are biologically unique, our systems metabolize and absorb foods at different rates. The amount and action of enzymes in breaking down food substances varies from individual to individual and at different ages of life. Emotional and psychological stresses of living have been shown to drive people into excesses of eating. Energy losses also vary depending on life style, occupation, and our individual physiological systems.

In keeping with the general idea of this entire book, my solution to the problem of excess weight is to try to simplify the approach. Perhaps I'm old-fashioned in this regard, but, in my opinion, motivation is more important than the program or the menus. A simple, uncomplicated weight-reducing method with strong motivation will produce good results.

The dangers of excess weight have been well-publicized. I don't want to belabor the point by reciting all of the inherent dangers of carrying around too many pounds on our respective frames. Let's consider just one aspect—the cardiovascular system. Excess weight places a strain on this most vital of systems. Treat your heart and accompanying blood vessels kindly by not imposing a weight burden on them. If you do take care of them by maintaining a sensible weight, the cardiovascular system will give you good and faithful service.

Dr. Daro's COSS System for Taking Off Weight

I don't have any miracle or revolutionary weight-reducing system to give you. Instead, I have something simple, effective, and uncompromising. All it does is ask the main purchasing agent or food buyer of the family not to bring home fattening foods, snacks, candy, cookies, pies, high-calorie sodas, ice cream, and desserts to the exclusion of or at the expense of nutritious, high-protein foods. That's it. If they're not there, you can't eat the junk foods. And, as suggested in a prior paragraph, the task is made easier today by the wide availability of many low-calorie food choices.

To sum up the whole Daro system for taking off weight, remember the acronym, COSS, which means *Cut Out Sugar and Starch.*

There's just one other simple element of the Daro reducing program, and that's exercise. I am not a stickler on the type of exercise that should be done or for how long. I don't lay out a program for my patients of so many pushups to be done or miles of jogging to be completed, and urge complete and blind adherence. When I have done this in a small way, I have found that more often than not people will start such a program with enthusiasm, and just as suddenly drop it after a few weeks. Too rigid a program invites rebellion. Walking, roller skating, indoor calisthenics, stretching, bicycling, jogging, golfing, tennis, volleyball—any of these activities or any other reasonably active form of exercise are fine. Do engage in any form of physical activity that you like but *do it daily!*

Many people try jogging because it's the "in" thing to do. Then, they find they don't like jogging, stop doing it, and subsequently end up not doing anything at all. They're afraid not to do the popular craze that is sweeping the country. My advice is to stick to some form of physical exercise that you truly enjoy rather than try to indulge in every new fad that come along.

Overweight Mother Changes Nutritional Habits and Loses 25 Pounds

A 38-year-old mother of four children who was approximately 30-35 pounds overweight requested that I put her on a special diet and prescribe some medication so that she could start to lose weight. I had to veto both ideas. The special diets are virtually useless for the reasons previously discussed. I don't prescribe pills because they only create a temporary and artificial situation for the user. Once they are discontinued, it's too easy for the individual to revert to previous bad habits.

I asked the patient if she were the one who bought food for the family. When I received her affirmative reply, I pointed out that weight reduction starts with what you select and buy in the supermarket. Because she was a mother, I reinforced the idea that through her example she was setting the pattern for the future health of her children. Because she was a wife, I cautioned her that by bringing home the wrong kinds of foods, she could be setting the stage for a heart attack or stroke for her husband. Basically, then, by appealing to her role as a mother, wife, and homemaker, I tried to solve her own weight-reducing problem, as well as having her build a sound nutritional program for her family. Obviously, what would be good for her in reaching her weight-loss goals would, simultaneously, have a beneficial effect for her family.

While she had come in seeking a "quick fix" for her overweight problem, I was able to convince her that the responsibility really was hers. She readily understood what I explained about using her judgment in selecting foods at the supermarket. She agreed with me that it made sense to establish the foundation of good health for her children, her husband, and herself. Fortunately, she was the kind of individual who accepted responsibility and the challenge I had thrust upon her. Our agreement was that she would report for monthly checkups.

This woman became the type of success story that I like to tell and write about. Her record of weight loss was as follows:

first month	7 pounds
second month	4 pounds
third month	4 pounds
fourth month	3 pounds
fifth month	2 pounds
sixth month	5 pounds
Total	25 pounds

I am not going to kid you by reporting that all my patients respond as well as this lady. The people that I have the greatest success with are those who like to assume responsibility for their own health. It usually turns out that these are the types of people who read health-oriented publications and books. They are strong believers in the philosophy that they can do as much as the medical profession in keeping themselves healthy if they have the proper guidance. They understand that they are the primary guardians of their own bodies.

I've told you how I have been able to help obese, married women. Now, what about single parents or the single individual? How and where do those of you in this category derive or develop motivation?

The key is creative selfishness. You have to learn to look out for the health of "Number One" which is *you*. What you are able to do, how you feel, and how you look need to be examined critically, and from there you must establish goals for self-improvement. While it may seem outwardly and completely selfish to be so concerned about *you*, in fact you will really be helping society as a whole. If we accept the premise that being overweight imposes health problems and that normal weight lessens the possibility of sickness, we, in effect, contribute to the overall health of society.

The most important motivation for losing weight is paying attention to how you feel carrying those extra pounds. Extra weight, as mentioned previously, imposes strain on all your bodily systems and, most of all, on your heart. Weight reduction for the obese will pay dividends far greater than any bank or savings institution can pay. As you reduce the load on your cardiovascular system, you will automatically have benefits credited to your health account. It's a guaranteed return.

Again, the formula is simple: COSS. *Cut Out Sugar and Starch.* Then exercise—moderately at first, but always consistently. It's better to walk around the block faithfully each evening than try to sprint 100 yards once or twice a week.

Chapter 12

Clogged Arteries

Bypassing the Bypass

In mentioning the next case, I am not suggesting that individuals receiving a diagnosis of clogged heart or coronary arteries should immediately reject the coronary bypass operation if it is recommended. The decision as to whether to go ahead with the operation or not is one that, obviously, requires all kinds of input—age, risk, physical condition, mental outlook, and medical alternatives. The subject should be thoroughly discussed with your doctor and the cardiologist before a final decision is reached. Having confidence in your medical advisers is as important as any other factor in the success of the operation and subsequent postoperative recovery.

How Nutritional Therapy Helped One Woman Bypass the Bypass

One of my long-time patients is a lady who is now 70 years of age. Five years ago she came in complaining of recurring chest pains and, also, a radiating pain down the upper part of her left arm. This could indicate a heart muscle that is being deprived of oxygen. If so, the coronary arteries that carry blood to the heart were probably clogged. Less blood with less oxygen was reaching the heart causing it to work harder and harder. Just as with any muscle deprived of oxygen, the heart gets a cramp and the individual suffers sharp pain. While you can massage a muscle or apply heat to bring more blood and relieve the spasm, therapy for a cramped heart muscle is not as easy, and, more importantly, therapy is much more critical.

I referred the patient to a cardiologist who admitted her to a hospital where an arteriogram was performed. An opaque fluid is injected into the coronary arteries and visualization by x-rays allows the arterial flow pattern to be studied. The original diagnosis of reduced flow in the coronary arteries was confirmed. It was recommended to the patient that she have a coronary bypass operation.

My patient is a feisty lady and simply refused to go ahead with the operation. She asked me if we could work something out on a nutritional basis to help with the condition.

We started by eliminating as many saturated fat components as possible from her diet. Butters, margarines, pies, pastries, cakes, gravies, and snack foods were put on the: "use sparingly, if at all, list." Lean meat, fish, vegetables, fresh fruit, and high-fiber cereals and breads were emphasized. The reason for the high fiber was to be certain that elimination would be a normal process and that there would be no straining that could increase the load on the heart. As part of the program to insure easy elimination, it was recommended that she drink a lot of water—six to eight glasses a day—in order to keep the stools soft. Caffeine-containing substances were also reduced in order to reduce overstimulation of the heart muscle until such time as our other therapeutic measures had time to take effect. A multivitamin-mineral supplement was included in the dietary program. In addition, I prescribed a chelated magnesium tablet—chelated to insure better absorption and utilization by the body. Next, I prescribed the liberal use of lecithin—the effective fat scavenger. I recommended to the patient that she take two to three tablespoons at least three times a day in whatever form she found most practical—sprinkled on a cereal, in a drink of orange juice, or any other method. Because of this lady's demonstrable strong will, I knew that she would stick to our plan of therapy.

It's been approximately five years now since she received the news of the diagnosis of obstructed coronary arteries and the recommendation for bypass surgery. She tells me that she has never felt better since starting the therapy described in the foregoing.

Again, I want to advise anyone who has received the same diagnosis not to immediately reject having the surgery done. Keep all of your options open and make any decision on the basis of obtaining as many facts as possible. If circumstances allow, seek out second and third opinions.

Another case in much the same situation was the husband of a patient. He, too, received a similar diagnosis. However, he elected to have the bypass surgery performed. He came to me at his wife's suggestion afterwards with the idea that he wanted to insure that there would be no recurrence of the clogging of the coronary arteries.

We prescribed the very same dietary and nutritional supplementation plan as for the lady. Interestingly, the two people became patients of mine at roughly the same time. He, too, reports feeling well from following the therapy. He says that he simply likes the feeling of assurance that he is helping the heart along by not imposing possible burdens or hazards from a bad diet or poor eating habits.

I want to point out that persons who have a bypass operation are not guaranteed a trouble-free existence from then on. If they do not alter dietary patterns and lifestyle, the same clogging of the new blood vessels that have been put into place can occur.

Studies show that approximately ten years after the operation, about half the patients who have had a bypass will have a return of chest pain. Studies also indicate that about two percent of all vein grafts close off each year in the first five years after surgery. In the next five years, the rate of closure increases to about five percent per year.

Is it not good preventive medicine, then, on your part to avoid the kind of diet that can place you in the position where one of the alternatives is having bypass surgery?

Start now to eliminate fatty foods from your diet. Eat generous amounts of fresh fruit and vegetables. Emphasize whole grain foods in your diet. Eat very lean cuts of meat. Order fish. Don't smoke. Cut out alcoholic drinks.

You'll help yourself bypass the bypass.

Chapter 13

Low Blood Sugar

The subject of hypoglycemia, or low blood sugar, is steeped in controversy. Some medical scientists say that it exists but is not very common. Others claim that there are approximately 40 to 50 million people who have it in various degrees of severity—ranging from a constant to a temporary hypoglycemic condition. Personally, based on my experience, I believe that it is more common than is generally thought by most physicians. I believe that consuming increasing amounts of sugar can wear out the body's ability to cope with and metabolically process it through various bodily systems. Just as you can overdose with aspirin, water, or milk, so obviously you can overdose with sugar.

One view of what happens in hypoglycemia is that there is a resulting malfunctioning of the pancreas. Blood sugar is regulated by insulin, which is produced by cells in the pancreas called the islets of Langerhans. A high consumption of sweets and starches is thought to overload the islets of Langerhans and cause a breakdown in the way insulin is released into the blood stream.

In my practice I find that patients referred to me will have had a complete battery of tests with the exception of the test specific for hypoglycemia. For example, the SMA includes 12 analytical determinations, including blood sugar, liver function, kidney function, cholesterol, and others. But, by itself, it does not provide the information necessary to detect hypoglycemia. The glucose tolerance test is the one that is specific for the purpose of determining hypoglycemia.

Glucose Tolerance Test

The procedure for the test is as follows: For three days, the patient eats a high-carbohydrate diet. On the fourth day, while the patient is in a fasting state, a blood sample is taken. The sugar level is determined. Next, the patient drinks a high-sugar-content liquid. Then, every hour for five hours, the blood sugar level is analyzed. In hypoglycemia, the blood sugar does not increase at the normal rate. It may happen that the initial rise due to the consumption of the high-sugar liquid is followed by a drop to below-fasting levels.

Effect of Low Blood Sugar

Brain cells are dependent upon blood sugar or glucose for nourishment. When there is a deprivation of glucose, the brain can be the first organ of the body to feel the effect. As a result of this phenomenon, the symptoms of hypoglycemia are most often associated with the nervous system. Studies demonstrate that people suffering from alcoholism, neurosis, and other neurological problems often have an underlying low blood sugar condition.

The problem with diagnosing hypoglycemia and the reason why it is often missed is that its symptoms mimic those of psychoneurotic conditions. These include: depression, irritability, anxiety, fears, difficulties in concentration and width of memory span, unjustified weeping, insomnia, fatigue, inability to make decisions, sensitivity to slight noise, and temper tantrums. All or some of these complaints may be complicated by sexual frigidity, nightmares, shortness of breath, dizziness, blurred vision, and thoughts of suicide.

With this array of symptoms and complaints, it is little wonder that physicians do not routinely order the glucose tolerance test. If a patient recites some of these complaints, the average physician has to believe that he has a full-fledged psychoneurotic on his hands. Thus, it's understandable that the first course of treatment might include tranquilizers, with little thought being given to changing the dietary habits of the patient. The mood-altering drugs, unfortunately, do little about the underlying causes of the hypoglycemic condition.

My Experience in Treating Hypoglycemia

If I suspect hypoglycemia and the glucose tolerance test comes back positive for the condition, I start a course of treatment that is simple and effective. I use the word "effective" guardedly here because I need the cooperation and commitment of the patient for the treatment to work. And, importantly, it's a natural approach because no medication or drugs are involved.

First, however, I want to point out one error in deduction that might occur. Because the blood sugar is low, it might be assumed that consuming more sugar and starches would solve the problem. This is wrong. Increasing the intake of sugar triggers the pancreas to manufacture more insulin with the result that the sugar level is depressed even more. The symptoms can worsen for the patient.

Therapy relies on the following approach:

1. Increased consumption of protein
2. Reduced amount of carbohydrates consumed
3. Eating smaller meals more frequently

My dietary recommendations include: fish, poultry, lean meats, eggs, cheese, fresh vegetables, fresh fruit, fresh fruit juices, milk, and plenty of water. If there is a taste need for coffee or tea, I recommended the decaffeinated types.

In preparing meat, poultry, and fish, I advise broiling, baking, or roasting. It is best to avoid frying. Because certain cuts of beef may prove economically burdensome in these inflationary times, chicken and tuna are comparatively inexpensive and very nutritious. Cheese and eggs are excellent sources of protein.

I do not recommend canned fruit and fruit drinks because they are overloaded with sugar. Oranges, grapefruit, apples, pears, peaches, nectarines, cantaloupe, berries, and watermelon are all on my recommended diet list.

Among the fresh vegetables an individual might select from are cauliflower, broccoli, green beans, carrots, lettuce, asparagus, tomatoes, and spinach.

I advise the hyoglycemic patient to avoid pies, cakes, puddings, cookies, crackers, popcorn, potato chips, sweet rolls, donuts, candy, pizza, pretzels, white bread, and pastas. Also taboo are wines, beer, cocktails, cordials, and sugared soft drinks. As mentioned a few paragraphs back, beverages with caffeine—tea, coffee, cocoas, colas—should be avoided because caffeine stimulates the liver to pour glucose into the blood stream. This produces the same bad effect caused by taking sugar.

I prefer the hypoglycemic patient to eat smaller meals with inbetween snacks or beverages to tide the patient over. The snacks can consist of a slice of cheese, small portion of cottage cheese, an apple or orange, a glass of milk, a handful of soybeans. By following such a dietary pattern, the hypoglycemic's blood sugar level is kept at a fairly even level. If there is too long a period between the ingestion of food, what may happen is a precipitous drop in blood sugar and the heightening of the unwanted and troublesome symptoms.

Fructose and Hypoglycemia

Fructose is an ideal food for the hypoglycemic person. In contrast to glucose, fructose is slowly absorbed from the digestive tract and doesn't accumulate to a high concentration in the blood. Where glucose at high concentrations in the blood stimulates the secretion of insulin, fructose does not. While pure fructose is expensive, I do recommend it to hypoglycemic patients who need a sweetening effect.

America's Eating Habits

As the reader reviews my dietary recommendations for relieving the symptoms of hypoglycemia, the perceptive observer of America's eating habits will be struck by the fact that a large majority of people eat items in the categories that should be avoided. Little children, teenagers, and adults make lunch time meals out of an order of french fries, hot dogs, coffee, or a cola drink. Breakfast might consist of a sweet roll and a cup of coffee for a large number of adults. Youngsters rely on cereals that are more sugar than whole grains. Is it any wonder, then, that many believe as I do, that hypoglycemia is far more prevalent than believed by many in the medical field.

Here are a few cases from my files illustrating what I have learned about treating hypoglycemia.

Dizziness, Blackouts, and Nervousness Disappear after Nutritional Therapy

The first case concerns a female patient, 22 years of age. Her principal complaint was that she had spotted the previous month. I ordered a thyroid test thinking that, perhaps, her symptom might indicate an underactive thyroid. However, the thyroid results came back normal. In the meantime, I prescribed a multiple vitamin-mineral supplement and vitamin B-complex tablet. To help relieve the spotting condition, I prescribed vitamin C.

Initially, the slight uterine bleeding seemed to be the primary complaint. Further interviewing, however, disclosed symptoms of dizziness, blackouts, nervousness, and a number of the symptoms associated with the hypoglycemic condition. Because of this combination of additional complaints, I ordered a six-hour glucose-tolerance test. I really wasn't surprised when the test results showed low blood sugar.

We provided the young lady with a high-protein, low-carbohydrate dietary program as outlined on the preceding pages. When she came in for periodic checkups, she reported that her symptoms had lessened and that her overall physical condition had improved. The dizziness, blackouts, and nervousness disappeared.

Irritability Relieved with Dr. Daro's Treatment

The next case is that of a 53-year-old female who was referred to me by another physician. Her complaint was that of bleeding, and an examination revealed a fibroid of the uterus. She was operated on and the uterus was removed. During the course of her postoperative visits to the office, the patient started to complain of dizziness, irritability, anxiety, lack of sex drive, and exhaustion. The combination of symptoms again strongly suggested a hypoglycemic condition and the glucose tolerance test was ordered. At the fifth hour, the blood-sugar level dropped below her fasting sugar level and confirmed the hypoglycemia. The patient was given the high-protein, low-carbohydrate diet. After a few weeks she reported that she was still experiencing periods of exhaustion throughout the day. I advised her to have additional snacks once, twice, or three times a day—as often as might be needed to combat the periods of physical letdown. Within three months, all of her symptoms had virtually disappeared. She reports that as long as she watches her diet, she has no further problems. In her case, I should add, that I made a vitamin B-complex tablet an integral part of the treatment, specifically to overcome the exhaustion problem.

Neurotic Complaints Virtually Eliminated after Nutritional Treatment

The third case is that of a female who has been a patient of mine for over 30 years. During that period of time, she always had a long series of neurotic complaints. I must admit that I simply was not aware then as I am now of the possibilities of hypoglycemia being the underlying cause. I ordered a glucose-tolerance test and the report came back showing a definite drop in blood-sugar level during the fourth hour. However, now, with the proper diet and supplementation with multivitamins and minerals, she is experiencing fewer of the neurotic symptoms. This has been a boon in all aspects of her life. She reports that her home life and relationship with her husband, children, and relatives has taken a decided turn for the better.

Most people, even if only marginally hypoglycemic, will derive many benefits from the dietary regimes I have outlined in this chapter. For the patients with the definite hypoglycemia, it has been like lifting a window shade to let the sun come in. Their symptoms disappear, their mental outlook turns around and they become new persons in many respects.

Chapter 14

Male Infertility

Being an obstetrician-gynecologist, my patients, obviously, are almost exclusively women. However, I have occasion to treat men, mainly because of the work I have been doing in the field of nutrition.

Of the problems affecting the space-age male, surprisingly, infertility is a disorder that appears with increasing frequency. Because we are alleged to be the best-fed country in the world, one would suppose that the male of the species would be receiving the proper nutrients in his daily meals to maintain his fertility.

As one might suspect, this is not the case at all in a number of instances. Improper dietary habits, overconsumption of alcohol, intemperate smoking, and, also, the use of drugs, in my opinion, are robbing many American males of their ability to reproduce.

Again, in my opinion, quite a bit of the problem can be traced to the fact that modern food processing removes so many vital nutrients in, for example, cereal grains. There is, of course, a commendable effort to return to the food product those valuable nutrients lost in the processing steps. In addition, we find more "natural" products now occupying the shelves of the supermarket.

Among the minerals that are lost in food processing is zinc. Zinc is vitally important in the development of secondary sexual characteristics and assumes a key role in the health and vitality of the male prostate gland.

Just a short aside here to illustrate how science catches up with nature and why supplementation remains a good idea. Man's need for zinc, according to one nutritional text, was not noted until 1961. This sequence is the usual scenario in the field of nutrition. Little by little scientific researchers note and identify roles for nutrient substances that are present in the natural, unadulterated, or fresh state of food. Unfortunately, the scenario has also shown that food processing has removed the nutrient before science has established its importance and role. The reinsertion of the nutrient in, perhaps, another form does not really compensate for its loss in the first place.

I wonder, also, about the statement in the same nutritional text that in the United States there is little danger of zinc deficiency. On the contrary, I would say there is a fairly good chance of zinc deficiency in a pretty easily definable segment of the population. These are the dieters and the poor eaters. We see them daily boarding commuter trains with a cup of coffee in one hand and a roll in the other.

Infertility Successfully Treated with Nutrition

One of the first cases of infertility that I treated was the husband of a patient of mine. The couple were anxious to become parents. The husband had consulted a urologist who advised that the husband's sperm count was too low and the activity of the sperm was insufficient. At this point the wife suggested to her husband that he consult with me for any ideas that I might have.

At first apperance there seemed to be nothing to suggest the cause for the husband's infertility. He was a vigorous young man of 27, who weighed 170 pounds and stood five feet ten inches tall. His overall physical condition was satisfactory. However, we could not deny that the laboratory analysis showed that the sperm count was low.

I suggested to the young man that he take a mineral-amino acid formulation. In addition to the broad spectrum of minerals and amino acids that it provided, I particularly wanted him to have zinc and arginine. Arginine has been classified as one of the semi-essential amino acids and I believe it to be important for increasing the sperm count and the motility of sperm. I also prescribed an additional zinc tablet for the young man. Zinc deficiency is associated with decreased function in male reproductive organs.

I suggested to him that he keep the course of treatment confidential for the time being. After following this course of treatment for a period of two months, I recommended that he visit the urologist and request another sperm test be done. The husband reported back to me that his sperm count had reached a normal level and that the urologist was amazed at the complete reversal of the condition. I might add that the couple were successful in becoming parents.

Rare Meat for Infertility

As I studied the problem of infertility, I became convinced that another precipitating factor might be the way in which food, especially meat, is prepared. As it happened, another case of infertility presented itself that allowed me to test the hypothesis.

The patient was a young man of 22 who was referred to me by another physician. This particular patient was slight of build, weighing 145 pounds, and five feet eight inches tall. The consultation produced the information that he relied heavily on snacks, pastries, cola drinks, and coffee for his nourishment. I learned that when he ate any steak, he always had it prepared well done. The report from the laboratory disclosed that his sperm count was only about 25 percent of normal.

I reoriented his entire dietary regimen and emphasized that he should eat plenty of eggs, cheese, seafood, and meat prepared rare. On a return visit he reported that he was following most of my recommendations and, particularly, that related to having his steaks and other beef dishes prepared rare. Because he was starting from a fairly run-down physical condition, I expected that any reversal that took place would take longer. The periodic checks that we did on the sperm count agreed with this forecast. Gradually, however, we noted that the sperm count did improve, and at the end of six months, there was a laboratory report showing that his sperm count was now normal.

This case led me to conclude that by eating rare meat, individuals can obtain a superior supply of amino acids. Very simply put, this is due to the fact that the amino acids are not subjected to excessive heat as in the case of well-done meats and, therefore, are not destroyed or diminished in the food-preparation process. Included in the amino acids available is, of course, the important arginine.

I want to point out here that there are other important sources of arginine, including: poultry, fish, calf's liver, peanuts, and peanut butter. In emphasizing beef steaks, I take into account the overall biologic value of the food product that means the availability of the other amino acids. In this regard, beef rates very high.

An Executive Regains His Fertility

A third case of treating sexual infertility involved an executive of a large multinational company. He was 33 years of age and while he and his wife were already the parents of two children, their efforts at producing a third conception had met with failure for a period of two years. His wife was a patient of mine and she spoke increasingly of the tension and frustration that she and her husband were experiencing. Because there seemed to be nothing wrong with her ovulatory process, I suggested that her husband come in to see me. As I anticipated, the laboratory tests showed the sperm count and motility to be below normal. During the consultation with the husband, I learned that as this young man climbed the corporate ladder of success, there were longer trips out of town with attendant problems in adhering to sound eating patterns. From what he told me I gathered there were increasing number of quick snacks and very often missed meals. In addition, he admitted to a higher consumption of alcohol and a heavier reliance on coffee and cola drinks.

Here again, the procedure was to reorient the patient to former, sound eating habits. I pointed out that his present dietary habits were undoubtedly robbing the cells of his reproductive system of the raw materials necessary for spermatogenesis. He agreed, and understood that a change in eating habits was necessary. I prescribed the amino acid-and-mineral combination formulation described previously along with an additional zinc tablet. Arginine, of course, was present in the combination formulation, along with other essential amino acids. I received his cooperation in getting back to sound eating habits with emphasis on fresh fruits and vegetables, milk, eggs, poultry, and meat. Since he already indicated that he liked to eat his meat rare, nothing was done in this area. I also strongly suggested that he cut down on his consumption of alcohol. Alcohol is a strong antagonist to many minerals and vitamins. On his fourth monthly visit, the laboratory report showed that his sperm count had returned to normal. One month later his wife became pregnant.

One of the reports that I received back from this patient and the other male patients is that the erection response improved, along with an apparent increase in penile size.

Sources rich in zinc are brewer's yeast, liver, shellfish, herring, pears, peas, egg yolk, beef, beets, sunflower seeds, mushrooms, milk, and wheat bran.

Vitamin C As an Aid in Infertility Cases

The lack of vitamin C has been associated with a condition called sperm agglutination which is a cause of male sterility. What happens is that sperm cells become sticky and clump together. When more than 25 percent of a man's sperm becomes stuck together in clumps, the male is unable to fertilize a female egg, according to one researcher.

At a meeting of the Federation of American Societies of Experimental Biology, Earl B. Dawson, a research associate professor at the University of Texas, Galveston, presented evidence that taking vitamin C supplements for one week can be enough to eliminate the problem.

In a research study, Professor Dawson compared two groups of men who had sperm agglutination problems and whose wives were not able to become pregnant. One group of men took placebo pills and a second group took vitamin C. In the space of just a few months, the wives of the men who were taking vitamin C became pregnant. None of the wives of the men who were given the placebo pills became pregnant.

Subsequently, Professor Dawson found an error in the study because the vitamin C that was supplied also had minerals that might have contributed to reducing the clumping or agglutination of the sperm cells.

In a follow-up study to correct the error, Professor Dawson supplied a group of male subjects who had a sperm agglutination problem with pure vitamin C. Then, sperm samples of these male subjects were analyzed at regular intervals. The researchers found in all cases that within seven days, the clumping or agglutination had reversed to a point where the sperm could fertilize an egg.

In order to verify the results, the researchers did another study in which they examined the sperm of a range of male subjects—some of the males were used as sperm donors while at the other extreme there were men with no viable sperm at all. They then analyzed the vitamin C level of the semen. From the data they saw a definite relationship between sperm cell clumping and vitamin C level. The higher the vitamin C level, the less clumping there was. And, the lower the vitamin C, the more agglutination they observed.

The male subjects in this study took one gram of vitamin C daily. The researchers point out that one glass of fresh orange juice daily would provide enough vitamin C to alleviate the problem.

Chapter 15

Skin Problems

The outer covering of the body receives more care, attention, and, perhaps, mistreatment than any other physiological system. The care is principally external and the covering, of course, is the skin.

While women receive most of the attention in advertising from cosmetic manufacturers and do most of the buying of deep cleansers, moisturizers, lipsticks, eye shadows, creams, oils, perfumes, sprays, and other skin products, men, also, are being catered to with increasing frequency. More and more cosmetic formulations directed to the male market are being developed, manufactured, and advertised.

With respect to the use of cosmetics, I think it appropriate to remind readers that in the not-too-distant past, many formulations could and did harm the skin and hair of many people. Some of the damage done was disfiguring and permanent. Presumably, today, the Food and Drug Administration is monitoring closely what goes into modern cosmetic formulas.

Hair and Skin as Health Signals

While cosmetics have a place in civilization as a means of embellishing appearance, too often people fail to see any connection between dietary habits and healthy, vital-looking skin and hair. Before applying chemical formulas to the skin and hair, isn't it a sound health practice to make sure first that a nutritional foundation has been established? It is interesting that veterinarians look at an animal's coat to judge its health. We, too, as humans should be conscious of the appearance of skin and hair in judging how well we are supplying our bodies with key nutrients.

The care of the skin involves more than just applying creams, colorings, and lotions from jars, tubes, and bottles. Beauty and health cannot come from external treatments. It has to begin from within.

The Three Nutritional Keys to Glowing, Healthy Skin

In my clinical experience, I have identified certain nutritional factors that prove beneficial in treating certain skin problems. For example, when I see dry, rough skin, I suspect a vitamin deficiency. I look for additional confirming signals, such as difficulty in adjusting to oncoming lights when driving at night. If the individual is a nondriver, I try to ascertain if there is sensitivity to sunlight or the reflected glare from other light sources. By now you might have determined that I am referring to a possible deficiency of vitmin A. In addition to these rather apparent clinical symptoms, we are able to confirm a vitamin A deficiency in the laboratory by means of a blood serum test.

Vitamin A Supplementation

The treatment for dry, rough skin that I have used successfully is supplementation with 25,000 to 30,000 units of vitamin A daily. In this type of treatment it is important to take some form of fat—butter, safflower oil, etc.—in order for this fat-soluble vitamin to be effective. Any kind of fat or oil stimulates the production of bile and it is this bile that protects the vitamin A from being destroyed.

Fat and Dry Skin

There are other conditions of dry skin that cannot be traced to a vitamin A deficiency. Another line of discovery I follow here is to determine the intake of fat on the part of the patient. I don't mean to imply that a heavy consumption of fat is necessary to combat a dry skin problem. However, a moderate amount of fat as present in polyunsaturated vegetable oils, for example, can contribute to improving, internally, the texture and feel of the skin. The softness and suppleness of the skin originates with the oils coming from the sebaceous glands. These, in turn, derive their raw materials from the fat content of our diets. Without some intake of fat, our skins would become dry and parchment-like. This is what happens to some people who severely restrict their fat intake. Conversely, by ingesting a moderate amount of fat, the individual is also contributing to the vitamin A intake; fats are sources of vitamin A. In this manner two nutrients important in combating dry skin are being made available to the body's metabolic processes.

Effect of Thyroid Gland on Skin Conditions

The other factor that figures in dry skin conditions is the thyroid gland. The symptoms that identify an underfunctioning thyroid gland include dry skin, cold hands, cold feet, exhaustion, and, sometimes, acute constipation. Treatment with thyroid alleviates the dry skin problem, as well as the other symptoms.

These three nutritional factors—vitamin A, fat, thyroid compound—if properly used with the guidance of a nutritionally knowledgeable physician can alleviate a majority of dry skin problems. Women and men spend millions of dollars on creams, ointments, and other oily formulas to lubricate their skin. Sometimes this type of treatment is important and necessary. The skier skiing down a slope into a cold and biting wind needs protection on exposed skin surfaces. Similarly, the outdoor worker, hunter, or even the salesperson making outside calls can use supplemental help to ward off the effects of wind, sun, or cold. However, it is also important where dry skin is a problem to be sure to take care of the body's own protective mechanism that can be brought into play. By treating from within, the body's own internal chemical reactions and lubrication processes are stimulated into activity.

On occasion I have also found that supplementation with the vitamin B complex also contributes to alleviating dry skin.

A Balanced Diet and Your Skin

It is important to stress that, in my experience, the dietary factors mentioned—vitamin A, fat, and thyroid—always work best when used in coordination with a balanced diet. The three factors are not magic elixirs to be used by themselves. The cells of the body need the minerals, vitamins, amino acids, protein, and liquid intake that only a well-planned and carefully followed diet can provide. You cannot rely on vitamin A alone, for example, to help with a dry skin problem and neglect to eat soundly. Don't expect vitamin A to be of assistance if you subsist solely on coffee, soft drinks, donuts, and french fries.

Just to review, if you have a meat, poultry, or fish entree, include a cooked vegetable, fresh vegetable salad, whole wheat bread for its fiber content, and a dessert of fruit instead of a piece of pie or cake. In addition, be sure to include as part of your dietary planning a multivitamin-and-mineral formula and eight glasses of water daily.

Now, it may seem odd that the nutritional factor that has a positive effect on dry skin problems also seems to help skin conditions having as their cause an excess of oil. However, in my experience, I have found that I can treat both kinds of problems with the same nutritional factor.

Vitamin A Helps Cure Sebaceous Cysts

One of my female patients, 55 years of age, came in with the skin on her back covered with several unsightly sebaceous cysts. And, she reported, that they were increasing in size. The inherent danger of these cysts is that they do grow larger in size if untreated and are susceptible to infection if they break open. The larger they become, the easier it is for rubbing against clothing or furniture, or scratching them, to cause them to break.

I prescribed the use of 30,000 units of vitamin A daily, along with attention to sound meal planning. Over a period of four months the condition gradually started to clear up. I must emphasize that the response time varies because of biological individuality. In cases of this kind, it can take from three to nine months for improvement to be noted. Vitamin A is not a "quick fix" by itself for a skin condition.

Another interesting case where vitamin A proved effective was that of a female, 45 years of age, who had a sebaceous cyst of the eyelid. When she first consulted me, she asked to be referred to an eye surgeon. I said that before we take that step, let's see if we can't treat from within with vitamin A. I estimated the size of the cyst at the beginning of therapy to be about ⅝″ in diameter. I started her on a course of vitamin A therapy and, of course, made certain that she understood about accompanying the vitamin A with some form of fat. After six months of this treatment, the cyst was barely perceptible.

How Vitamin A and Zinc Cleared Up Teenager's Acne

Another condition that responds fairly well to vitamin A therapy is acne. In addition, I have found that vitamin A and zinc work well together in treating acne. The results are better than using just one of the nutrients.

One case was that of a very pretty 19-year-old college student who was experiencing a mild depression because of a rather severe case of acne. She was extremely self-conscious and complained that her social activities and life were restricted as a result. Young people, of course, suffer the most when acne affects parts of the body that are not covered by clothing. This young lady's face and forehead were severely affected with acne and she, also, had the sores on her chest and back. In her case I decided that a combination of vitamin A and zinc in the form of zinc gluconate would be the basis of her treatment. I also pointed out the necessity of cutting down on the consumption of hydrogenated fats as contained in french fries, margarine, and potato chips. The dosages I recommended in her case were 25,000 units of vitamin A and 45 mg. of zinc gluconate. I saw her every two weeks and, within a span of three months, her acne condition cleared up and her depression lifted.

Acne vulgaris is common to oily skin and occurs most frequently on the face, chest, and back. While usually associated with adolescence, it may occur at any age. It is an inflammatory disease of the sebaceous or fat glands that results when the fatty secretions are blocked from release. Blackheads then form and become very unsightly.

One interesting case in my experience was that of a very prominent surgeon in Chicago who had had a very severe case of acne for many years. Being part of the medical profession he, of course, had access to his medical colleagues for treatment and advice. Unfortunately, none of the practitioners he consulted had any interest in or knowledge of nutritional forms of therapy. He heard about some of my work and came to see me. His back was covered all over with acne. There was not a square inch of his skin that was free of the sores. I suggested that he take 15 mg. of zinc in the form of the gluconate three times a day. He was skeptical but having tried everything else, he agreed to follow the therapy. A few months later when I looked at his back, the acne was completely gone. He was extremely happy with the results because he was now able to participate in many more activities such as swimming without the acute embarrassment that he felt previously. In addition, he has referred other patients with acne problems to me.

I have treated hundreds of cases of acne and the majority have experienced relief from either the vitamin A or zinc, or a combination of both.

Help for Psoriasis

Psoriasis is a chronic skin disease that attacks both the young and the old. It is characterized by red spots on the skin that are covered with a silvery scale. Because of the unsightliness of these lesions, it obviously has a destructive effect psychologically on the sufferer. Persons afflicted with psoriasis will often resort to a number of strategies to avoid exposing his or her skin to view. They seek to avoid sports or athletic activities where it becomes necessary to expose parts of the anatomy. For example, they may stay away from swimming completely, even though it may be a favorite activity. Or, even where the sport may not entail a great deal of body exposure, they will not participate because they have to take off their street clothes in a locker room in order to change into a sweat or workout suit. In other words, their lives may become quite restricted because they do not wish to show other people the skin lesions they have to live with.

It is revealing to read texts on nutrition and disease and find that they dismiss vitamins and diet as being of little help in alleviating the symptoms of the disease. Unfortunately, medical professionals are exposed to these texts and may develop biases that prevent them from evaluating different methods of therapy. Patients with psoriasis who consult with physicians often become discouraged and frustrated at the lack of progress being made in the treatment of this very annoying disease.

85-Year-Old Psoriasis Victim Improved through Better Nutrition

One of the oldest psoriasis sufferers I had as a patient was a gentlemen 85 years of age. His was a most severe case. His entire body was covered with the unsightly red spots—face, arms, hands, chest, back, legs, and feet. There was scarcely one inch of his skin that was free of the blemishes. When he first consulted with me, he said that he had been to a number of leading dermatologists without obtaining any long-term relief. Quite naturally he was discouraged at what the medical profession had thus far provided for him.

The key to treatment-Lecithin. Contrary to what the texts on nutrition have to say on the matter, I devised a program of diet, multivitamins and minerals, vitamin A, vitamin E, vitamin C, and a key component of the plan, lecithin. The actual food part of my program emphasized fresh fruits and vegetables, protein, whole grain cereals and bread, and deemphasized carbohydrates, cakes, pies, cookies, candy, white bread, rolls, potato chips, and similar empty-calorie foods. I recommended that he take a tablespoon of lecithin four times a day. Lecithin can be sprinkled on cereal, salad, or mixed in juices and other beverages. A theory regarding the cause of psoriasis is that it results from a disturbance in fat metabolism. Lecithin is a phospholipid and the phospholipids play very important roles in metabolism. They are compounds in cell membranes, essential parts of certain enzyme systems, and involved in the transport of fats in the body.

Lecithin's Detergent-Like Action. Lecithin is the most abundant of the phospholipids in body tissues and foods. Lecithin, I believe, acts as a biologic detergent with specific reference to solubilizing lipids or fatty materials. In effect, I believe it works to wash out fatty materials. At least I am convinced of this based on the results it has produced in the treatment of psoriasis.

Within three months my 85-year-old patient was completely free of the lesions of psoriasis. He was more than overjoyed because he had never in his entire life experienced relief of this nature before. To the present time he has had no recurrence of the problem. He continues with the multivitamin and minerals, sound diet plan, and, of course, the lecithin.

A second case concerned a 55-year-old woman who came to me complaining of the characteristic lesions of psoriasis which, as in the previous case, covered her entire body. She told me that she had had the affliction for 35 years and had visited dermatologists and other specialists without any long-lasting relief. In cases of this kind, the conventional treatment consists of salves and ointments. The patient complained of the messiness involved in applying the ointments and, of course, the ensuing problems with trying to keep clothing clean.

I interrogated her regarding her diet. It was deficient in the areas I regard as important in combating psoriasis.

I directed her to a diet high in protein—fish daily, lean meats, poultry, and nuts. In addition, the diet plan included vegetables, either raw or lightly cooked, and fruit. I also noted that she did not drink enough liquids and I emphasized that she should have water and fresh fruit juices to the extent where her total volume would approximate two quarts of liquid daily.

I prescribed: lecithin, four tablespoons daily; vitamin E, 800 units daily; and vitamin C, 3,000 mg. daily. To this was added a multivitamin-and-mineral formulation. In addition, she was advised to eliminate margarine and butter and in their place to use safflower oil—at least four tablespoons daily. The safflower oil is for use on salads or eggs, or in frying foods.

Her conditioned cleared up in approximately four months and in the intervening months, her skin has remained dry. She has no complaint of itching and no longer has to use any ointments. She is very happy with the results we were able to achieve.

Vitamin E Helps Healing Process

Two recent cases that I have been treating both involve males. The first is that of a man, 67 years of age, who has been bothered with psoriasis on his derriere and elbows. According to the medical history I have on the patient, he has had the problem for some 50 years. I am following the same therapeutic regime—diet with emphasis on protein, vitamins A, E, and C in the amounts as previously outlined, and lecithin. Because I know of its benefits in treating burn tissue, I am adding another factor. I am using vitamin E oil directly on the lesions to determine if this will hasten the healing process. I have been encouraged by the fact that new skin is appearing on the circumference of the lesions. As pointed out in the previous cases, the therapy is not a quick cure. The effect of diet modification takes time to take hold. Years of poor eating habits are not altered overnight. We are seeing results and the patient is experiencing a change in his psychological outlook which is an extra benefit I always look forward to seeing.

The fourth case is that of a young man of 20 years of age. His back and chest are covered with the psoriasis and, of course, this has provided a detriment to certain athletic interests and activities. He has been afflicted with the condition for some seven years. Our approach, as before, uses diet reorientation, vitamins A, E, and C, lecithin, and the multi-vitamin-and-mineral formula.

How Nutrition Can Help Counter Damaging Effects of the Sun

Moderate exposure of the skin to the sun done slowly and carefully can produce a nice, healthy-looking tan; and, of course, vitamin D is generated in the body by exposure to sunlight. However, continued overexposure of the skin to the sun can lead to many problems. The skin can become very dry and brittle due to the loss of natural oils and lead to premature aging of the skin. Even more serious is the possible development of skin cancer.

Nature's Most Effective Sun-Screen

To protect the skin against the ravages of overexposure to the sun, I have found PABA, or para-aminobenzoic acid, a very effective screening agent. When the compound is used prophylactically, the skin does not redden and burn. Anyone sensitive to the sun would be wise not to risk exposing their skin without the protection afforded by PABA.

PABA is available either in lotion or cream form. In addition, it can be taken internally in a dosage of 250 mg., three times daily. The lotion can be used before and after exposure to the sun to obtain the maximum benefit from its action.

Entire Family Obtains Relief

One of my patients was a telephone operator who was the mother of two children. The family was about to start on a vacation trip to Florida. They were concerned because they were all fair skinned and had a long history of suffering from sunburn, even though they tried to minimize their outdoor exposure. In a sunny climate this is difficult even wearing protective clothing. While the direct rays of the sun may be avoided fairly successfully, there is always a considerable amount of reflected exposure from the shiny surfaces of cars, glass windows, water, and light-colored pavement.

I advised them to buy PABA lotion and, in addition, to take PABA orally as mentioned previously—250 mg. three times daily. They followed this preventive program and upon their return, they reported that they experienced no painful episodes of sunburn. This was the first time that they were able to truly enjoy a vacation in a sunny climate and they continue to follow this simple but effective routine.

Woman Able to Enjoy Sunshine Again

Another case was that of a patient 50 years of age who lives in Florida the year around. She was in Chicago visiting relatives who suggested that she come to see me. Like the people in the previous case, she had extremely sensitive skin and quite naturally had to control her outdoor exposure periods and wear long-sleeved dresses, slacks, and wide-brimmed hats. Shorts and short-sleeved blouses were out and this can pose quite a problem in the heat of Florida. Because of the sensitivity of her skin and the painful episodes of sunburn she had endured in the past, she often would limit her time in the outdoors to early morning and after sundown. This imposed quite a burden for she was naturally gregarious and had become almost a prisoner in her home.

I prescribed PABA lotion for external application to the skin and, also, PABA in the form of the 250 mg. tablets, three times daily. With this program she has been able to tolerate the sun more easily and has had fewer painful bouts of sunburn that would formerly lay her up for days. While she cannot expose her skin for too long a period of time to the direct rays of the sun, she is no longer so restricted in her activities nor in the type of outdoor clothing she can wear.

Bioflavonoids for Black-and-Blue Marks

Ecchymosis is a frightening word. However, it simply refers to the black-and-blue marks that may occur, for example, when you bump or strike some object. Some people are particularly vulnerable. This points up the phenomenon of biological individuality. Just as some of us may be more prone to ecchymosis, so may our individual biological systems require nutrients in different amounts. The underlying cause of ecchymosis is increased capillary fragility and permeability. In this situation I have been able to help patients through the use of bioflavonoids. I have found that having patients take between 500 to 1,000 mg. of bioflavonoids, three times daily, to be effective in ameliorating the condition.

Black-and-Blue Marks Disappear

A recent case is that of a close, personal friend of mine. He is a gentleman, 60 years of age, who was receiving cortisone therapy for an arthritic condition. His wife confided to me in a telephone conversation that her husband's skin was displaying black-and-blue marks with increasing frequency. She also mentioned that his physician was prescribing heavy doses of vitamin C. However, she said that this did not seem to be having any effect on the black-and-blue mark condition. I prescribed bioflavonoids and within two weeks the black-and-blue marks disappeared.

Vitamin C is essential for the production of intercellular material that strengthens the walls of the capillaries. Bioflavonoids function as antioxidants and protect vitamin C from oxidative destruction. The effect of bioflavonoids on the maintenance of normal capillary strength may be considered to be indirect by way of ascorbic acid.

Chapter 16

Female Problems

As an obstetrician-gynecologist, among the most common complaints I hear from women concern menstrual problems, including premenstrual tension, irregular flow, and missed periods. Other problems revolve around the use of birth control pills, menopause, and, while not a complaint as such, toxemias of pregnancy. I have been able to help women with these problems using a nutritional approach. Because there are different causes for these conditions, the diagnosis must, of course, confirm that there is or can be a nutritional deficiency. And, while not all patients respond equally, the positive results that I have obtained reinforce the idea that nutritional factors can help uncomplicate certain, natural, biological phenomena occurring in a woman's body.

The Link between Premenstrual Tension (PMS) and Nutrition

The menstrual period in modern societies, unfortunately, has come to be a medical problem of rather large proportions. There are, of course, many influencing factors as to why this has occurred. Part of the problem stems from the fact that we have imparted the idea to women that slight discomfort needs immediate medication or other attention. Certainly, you and your physician should be alert to deviations from the normal but, at the same time, this should be counterbalanced by the knowledge that if we treat our biological machinery with fairness—and, of course, I mean from the nutritional point of view—it will serve us well. It is reported that women in primitive cultures experience relatively short and uncomplicated menstrual periods. If this is partially related to the fact that they subsist on simpler, more basic diets, then, perhaps, there is a lesson here for women in more modern societies that a trip back to basics in eating habits may help relieve some menstrual problems and generally promote good health.

Premenstrual tension, or PMS as it is commonly called, is characterized by a wide-ranging group of symptoms. The condition can last from a few to several days prior to menstruation and continue right on into the menstrual period. Symptoms include: anxiety, irritability, mental depression, crying, and insomnia. Other signs are an edema or swelling of the breasts, abdominal cramping, constipation, weight increase, and headaches. In addition, resistance to infections can be at a low point. Women will experience some of these symptoms, and the severity and length of time involved, of course, determines how personally distressing the premenstrual problem is for each individual.

I do believe that, as part of the therapy, women can reprogram themselves mentally from the severity of particular symptoms. As the menstrual period approaches, if you say to yourself that you will have your "usual" headache, your body probably won't disappoint you. Conditioning yourself with and reinforcing positive ideas can help lessen the impact of various symptoms.

Menstruation should be symptom free in women who are meeting their nutritional requirements and who are without other infections or disease. It follows, too, that the premenstrual period should be without complication. In my practice, however, I have found that furnishing two minerals in particular seem to meet a deficiency need and help relieve PMS. However, as always, I believe that supplementation alone cannot solve the problem completely. As always, eating from the four basic food groups is the foundation for correcting imbalances and promoting good health. Vegetables, fruits, dairy products, protein sources, and whole grain foods are the price of admission to ameliorating premenstrual tension. Sweet rolls, heavily sugared cereals, salty snack foods, and similar empty calorie foods are out. In fact, women with swelling problems should avoid salty foods. Water fills tissue to counterbalance the effect of the sodium ion. In selecting foods making up the basic four, I suggest, if possible, foods rich in calcium and magnesium. These are the two minerals that I have found helpful in treating PMS. Below are some foods that are rich in calcium and magnesium.

Calcium	*Magnesium*
almonds	almonds
apricots, dried	apricots, dried
brazil nuts	beans, lima
broccoli	brazil nuts
buttermilk	bread
cereal, oat	rye
cheese	whole wheat
American	cashew nuts
Swiss	cereal
collards	cornmeal
dandelion greens	oat
figs, dried	shredded wheat
fish	chard, raw
salmon	cheese
sardines	cheddar
kale	parmesan
milk	coconut, shredded
skim	collards
whole	crackers, graham
molasses	dates, dried
mustard greens	figs, dried
soybean curd (tofu)	molasses
turnip greens	okra
yogurt	parsley
	peanuts, unsalted

Magnesium (cont'd)
soybean curd (tofu)
spinach
wheat germ

Blood calcium falls prior to menstruation and the lowered level can contribute to nervous tension and irritability. In addition, an inadequate amount of calcium seems to cause a retention of salt contributing to the swelling symptom. Magnesium is an essential element in human metabolism and is critical in the work of nerves and muscles. Its adequate supply in the diet thus contributes to producing a calming effect. It, too, seems to play a role in regulating the flow of sodium in and out of tissue.

I have found that, in addition to working out the details of a good diet for my patients with PMS and deemphasizing salt, I obtain good results with a calcium-magnesium tablet. I prefer prescribing a chelated product that seems to improve absorption. The preceding treatment routine has produced good results for hundreds of my patients. I know it works because I have also received telephone calls from many husbands of my patients expressing their thanks for their more tranquil wives.

No More Breast Tenderness and Swelling

A typical patient was a single parent, 31 years of age, who was an assistant buyer for a department store chain. A particular and long-standing complaint of hers was tender and swollen breasts. In consultation, we identified sources of salt in her diet and advised eliminating as much of this as possible. I prescribed four tablets daily of the chelated calcium-magnesium product to be taken approximately six to seven days prior to menstruation. She reported back to me that within a few months she no longer had episodes of tenderness and swelling of her breasts.

Premenstrual Irritability Relieved

Another patient was 27 years old, married, with two children. She was a referral from her family physician and she complained about headaches and irritability. She was alarmed at what the episodes were doing to her family life, as apparently she was getting into arguments with her husband with increasing frequency. She even admitted that she was entertaining throughts of running away. In delving into her dietary patterns, I found that she was eating and munching indiscriminately on a lot of junk foods—including many salty snacks. I convinced her that this salt buildup could produce headaches because the brain swelled just like any other tissue. We eliminated this food factor and gave her a dietary plan that was a complete reversal from what she was eating. I prescribed the chelated calcium-magnesium supplement, along with a total vitamin-mineral tablet. Subsequently, she told me that the number of headaches had virtually dropped to zero and, simultaneously, she lost some seven to eight excess pounds. She said that she was no longer irritable and that marital quarrels were less of a problem. Her husband called me and confirmed that what might have been a growing conflict had been averted.

Headaches Disappear

A third case was that of a 35-year-old supermarket checker with symptoms of insomnia, nervousness, and headaches. When I first saw her, she told me that she was taking up to six aspirins daily to relieve headache pain. When unable to sleep, she admitted to fixing herself a couple of martinis. The alcohol alone was compounding the problem by robbing her body of magnesium. I convinced her to give up snacking on candy bars, breakfasting on sweet rolls and coffee, and prescribed a multivitamin-and-mineral formulation, the chelated calcium-magnesium tablet, some extra vitamin C to help her fight colds to which she seemed to have little resistance, and based all of this, of course, on a major overhaul of her diet. Because of this patient's somewhat poorer nutritional status, it took a few months before she was able to feel relieved of her various symptoms. The headaches disappeared rather quickly. It was the insomnia that took a little longer period of time.

As a footnote to these cases, I feel that in treating such cases in this manner, with the chelated calcium-magnesium formulation, we might possibly be aiding a long-term development that afflicts women, in particular. This is osteoporosis. The demineralization of bone that occurs is attributable to the lack of calcium. Perhaps with this kind of supplementation, we are laying the groundwork for forestalling the development of this debilitating disease. Vitamin D is a necessary accompaniment to the utilization of calcium and is obtained, of course, rather easily through such vitamin D-fortified products as milk.

Irregular Menstrual Flow

There are a number of factors that can be involved in irregular menstrual flow including malnutrition, infection, increased exercise, and heightened sexual activity. An underactive thyroid gland may be responsible for profuse bleeding. If tests for determining the activity of the thyroid confirm this and there seems to be no other medical problems, I may recommend foods rich in iodine. Iodine is necessary for proper functioning of the thyroid. In rank order from high to low, foods containing iodine include seafoods, vegetables, meat products, eggs, dairy products, bread, cereals, and fruit. The closer the food is grown or raised to the coasts of oceans, the higher the iodine content. I have had some success with this approach.

On other occasions I have used extra supplementation with vitamin E to correct heavy bleeding problems. Added supplementation with iron is frequently necessary to compensate for its loss due to the excessive menstrual flow.

These conditions need close and careful diagnosis and attention by a physician who knows how and when to apply nutritional therapy if appropriate.

Bioflavonoids Correct Menstrual Bleeding Problem

My experience with bioflavonoids began with a patient whom I had delivered of three children. She came into the office about one year after the birth of her last child and complained of having bleeding problems. I prescribed the bioflavonoids in a dosage of 1000 mg., three times daily. I told her that if that didn't work, we would have to do a D and C (dilatation and curettage) to clean out the interior of her uterus. I didn't see her again for a few months until the time of her next checkup. She came in and spoke enthusiastically of how the bioflavonoids had checked the bleeding problem. She also added that two friends of hers had been scheduled to have curettements. On her recommendation they took the bioflavonoids. They, too, found that their bleeding problems were corrected and they did not have to undergo the D and C procedure. Obviously, anyone trying bioflavonoids and finding that the bleeding situation is continuing should not put off consulting with their personal physician. A fair trial for the bioflavonoids is approximately two to three months.

Nurse helped.

Interestingly, I told this story to a group of nurses at the outpatient clinic of Columbus Hospital in Chicago where I still do some private practice work. One of the nurses came to me about three months later and told me that because of my conversation with them, she started the bioflavonoids. She was very pleased with the results she obtained and said that her bleeding problem between periods had disappeared.

Missed Periods or Amenorrhea

The hormone-producing glands, like all tissues of the body, need proper nutritional support. The key or master gland is the pituitary. If you starve it, you affect its influence on the ovaries that produce estrogen. In turn, estrogens act to increase uterine flow.

With this pattern in mind, extreme starvation to shed extra pounds can produce a chain reaction throughout the body. I have had women as patients who have dieted strenuously and their menstrual periods cease. This brings to mind the case of an 18-year-old girl who was well developed and menstruating at the proper time, suddenly, concerned about becoming thin, having her menstruation stop. She was skipping breakfast, subsisting on a small sandwich for lunch and eating only the skimpiest of dinners—maybe a bowl of soup, cheese and crackers, or yogurt. She achieved a weight loss, but in the process, was inflicting havoc on all the cells and tissues of her body.

The solution to this case of amenorrhea was reorienting this young lady's thinking about the necessity of eating foods with nutritional value while at the same time helping her maintain the body weight she had fixed as an objective. I emphasized a high-protein diet with selections from fish, poultry, and lean cuts of beef. Carbohydrates were to be obtained principally from fresh fruit and vegetable sources and whole grain foods. I prescribed a multivitamin-and-mineral formulation along with extra vitamin C. Due to her lowered nutritional status, I wanted to help build up her resistance to infection and the extra vitamin C, I felt, provided this. In addition, I suspected that because of her crash diet, she would be low in iron. A simple blood test confirmed this and I emphasized that she eat liver and fish two or three times a week. These foods contain iron in the organic heme form, which the body absorbs more readily. This was a case where the results took a while to achieve because of the comparatively depleted state of the patient's biological system. It was necessary for her to come into the office regularly, so that I could monitor her progress carefully. Within three months, she improved to the point where she was back on schedule with her menstrual cycle.

Obviously, malnourishment, as in this case, is not the only cause of amenorrhea. Amenorrhea is not, by itself, a disease. Rather, it may be the symptom of a hormonal imbalance that may be temporary in nature, or a signal of something more serious. As a result the underlying causes may not be so readily treated and solved as happened in this case. But, if you do follow sound dietary patterns and supplementation with vitamins and minerals, it increases the chances of your not developing the problem initially, or coping with it more successfully. To give an illustration, cirrhosis of the liver can precipitate amenorrhea. Thus, if you don't drink alcohol, you most likely will not develop cirrhosis of the liver, which by itself is bad enough, and the chances of developing amenorrhea from this cause are minimal. There are congenital problems that good nutrition can't alter directly but can put you in a state of improved health to make such treatment as might be applied more successful.

Birth Control Pills Increase Need for Supplementation

Birth control pills vary in their formulation according to the estrogen and progesterone content and in the side effects that they produce. As might be expected, women of various ages and physical condition respond differently. Some of the side effects are relatively minor and, others, as has been well publicized, have serious and life-threatening consequences. Women electing to use birth control pills should also be aware that nutritional deficiencies can result. The use of birth control pills has been said to produce false pregnancy, and like a real pregnancy, a woman should furnish her body with proper and even extra nutrition.

I think it's worthwhile here to review and remind women who are on birth control pills what they face potentially and why, as a matter of good preventive medicine, they should keep themselves fit nutritionally.

There are a number of side effects that are referred to as minor, relatively speaking. For example, some women react to an excess of estrogen provided by the pill with nausea and vomiting. Dizziness and headaches are other reactions. Water retention can be a problem that then reflects itself by a swelling of the breast and legs. These problems should be referred to the prescribing physician as they occur.

Mental depression is a rather frequently reported side effect that is said to be due to an excess of progesterone provided by the pill. Fatigue and tiredness are other side effects that, reportedly, are due to progesterone excess. Where these symptoms appear, supplementary vitamins, particularly the B-complex group, can help alleviate the problem. Pyridoxine, vitamin B-6, is particularly helpful. Always, however, keep in mind that a sound diet is the starting point for obtaining the maximum benefit from any vitamin-mineral supplementation.

Decreased sex drive, oiliness of the skin, and acne are other side effects that may accompany birth control pills. The vitamin B-complex can be important here, too, in relieving the symptoms. Remember that the B vitamins work synergistically with each other and all are needed, as well as the rest of the ingredients of multivitamin and mineral formulations. What is being suggested here is that additional amounts of the B complex, above and beyond what is in a multivitamin-and-mineral formula, can possibly help...in consultation with and guidance from a medical professional.

Another condition that can result from taking birth control pills is a fungal or yeast infection called *monilia vaginitis*. It appears that the pills increase the glucose content of the cells of the vagina. This factor, along with other predisposing conditions in the vagina such as it being wet, warm, and dark, make the vagina a fertile breeding ground for the growth of a fungus. Diabetes and obesity are preexisting conditions that also contribute to the development of fungal infections. Nutritionally, with respect to this problem, women taking birth control pills, diabetics, and the obese would be well advised to severely limit or eliminate entirely those heavily sugared products in their diets. This is particularly true, of course, if you have a history of such fungal infections. Another thing that might be tried is to eat plain yogurt that has live cultures to counteract the yeast in the vagina. The actual treatment for monilia infection uses fungistats.

In the category of serious or major side effects are those involving the cardiovascular system.

Birth control pills increase the chances for developing blood clots by an estimated five to ten times. The sites for such blood clots include superficial or close-to-the-surface veins, and the deep-vein network of the legs. Clots occurring in the deep venous network are more serious and life threatening. Then, we have the possibility of cerebral thrombosis, or strokes, occurring in the brain with obvious dire consequences. Whether blood clots in the leg or cerebrovascular accidents, women taking birth control pills increase their chances for such occurrences particularly if they have pre-existing medical problems such as diabetes, obesity, hypertension, or vascular problems. Women who take the pill and continue to smoke are in double jeopardy as far as laying themselves open to a stroke.

Other serious complications resulting from birth control pills include heart attack, hypertension, and gallbladder disease.

As mentioned earlier in this section, nutritional deficiencies occur from taking the pill. The corrective action is to eat a diet emphasizing protein. You don't want to put on weight by consuming a lot of carbohydrates and edge yourself over into the higher risk group for cerebral or other blood-clotting accidents.

Drink extra amounts of water to wash through any excess sodium, thereby avoiding swelling or edema. Don't smoke.

Take a multivitamin-mineral formulation, additional B complex vitamins in the event of feelings of fatigue or depression, and extra vitamin C to build up your infection-fighting reserves. I also think that magnesium in the form of chelated calcium-magnesium can be helpful. Magnesium has been found to have a positive effect as far as blood clots are concerned. Likewise, vitamin E in additional amounts can serve as an anticoagulant. Again, consult with a medical professional who, hopefully, will have a nutritional background before trying such therapies on yourself.

Treatment for Symptoms of Menopause

Some statistics indicate that 75 percent of American women experience few if any of the symptoms of menopause. If you are in the remaining 25 percent, that is little comfort. However, if you are in that smaller group, it might be some small solace to know the symptoms of the change of life do wind themselves down after a few years. The lesser symptoms include hot flashes and sweating. The more serious symptoms include hysteria, constipation, heart pain, ulcers, and mental depression.

I have used vitamin E with good results in relieving hot flashes. While vitamin E is not as effective as estrogen replacement therapy, ERT, it does not have the inherent dangers.

Estrogen can, in excess, increase the possibility of uterine and breast cancer.

The best way that I know of meeting menopausal problems head on is through good nutrition and, also, not to condition yourself to expect the worst. Do not say to your physician or to a friend, "I understand that a woman in the menopause has to suffer through..." Do not reinforce the thought that something negative is going to happen. There are many books on the market that teach and guide one to develop positive attitudes. I would recommend reading books of this kind in the event that you might be approaching menopause with some trepidation. It's just as easy to learn to think positively as negatively and with the right mental perspective you can sail right on through this period of life without any storms whatsoever.

To place yourself in the best possible physical condition, pay close attention to your weight. Obviously, if you are closer to a normal weight, hot flashes will not be compounded by any extra burdens of excess weight on your cardiovascular system. Dietary supplementation with a complete formula of vitamins and minerals will maintain bone strength and energy that some women feel a loss of during the menopause. To fend off the development of osteoporosis, which is not necessarily related to the menopause but which can be getting a start about this time, eat plentiful quantities of green leafy vegetables that are rich in calcium. Drink whole or skim milk for the same reason. Drink copious quantities of water, preferably distilled, to flush out toxins and, additionally, avoid the problems of constipation. Keep active physically, even if it's only sit-ups, leg raises or walks around the block.

I do not like prescribing tranquilizers. If there are symptoms of nervousness, a glass of milk is still a pretty good way to calm nerves, promote relaxation, and induce sleepiness. In my own case, in the event I am having trouble sleeping, I have already mentioned that tryptophan, an amino acid, is helpful. It is involved in the production of serotonin in the brain, which is linked to our ability to fall and remain asleep. Prolonged intake of tryptophan may result in a deficiency of vitamin B-6. Thus, tryptophan is more effective when taken with vitamins B-6 and C, both of which are needed for its metabolism. In these efforts it is advisable to work with a knowledgeable and medically trained nutritionist.

Eclampsia—How Sound Nutrition Helps Avert This and Other Problems of Pregnancy

In the "Early Experiences" chapter in this book, I mentioned eclampsia as a problem that can affect pregnant women. There are, of course, a number of conditions, called toxemias of pregnancy, which can occur during a pregnancy. I am going to discuss eclampsia here in a little more detail because I have studied it and applied a lot of effort to preventing its occurrence. If allowed to develop, it has severe consequences for both the mother and the fetus, and I believe that close attention to the diet and nutrition of the pregnant woman is good preventive medicine with respect to eclampsia. On an even more positive note, there is no greater gift that a mother-to-be can bestow on her unborn child than good health, and nutritional preparation and build-up should occur way before conception, and continue right on into and through pregnancy.

Eclampsia

Eclampsia is divided into two stages—pre-eclampsia and eclampsia. I add a third stage where I find it most productive to initiate the preventive approach through diet and nutrition.

The symptoms of pre-eclampsia and eclampsia are similar and vary only in degree. They include, but are not limited to, hypertension, edema, albuminuria, and excessive weight gain. The most severe symptoms, coma and convulsions, occur in the eclamptic stage. Albuminuria refers to the presence of albumin in the urine. How serious is this whole syndrome? Pre-eclampsia has a maternal mortality of 1 to 2 per 1000 patients and fetal mortality of 10 per 1000 patients. If eclampsia develops, then the maternal mortality reaches 50 to 100 per 1000 cases and fetal mortality rises to 200 to 250 per 1000 cases.

Women who are at the greatest risk in developing eclampsia are those who are malnourished, young, and having their first baby. Also at high risk are those with hypertension problems, and diabetics.

Threatened Pre-Eclampsia

My study of the problem led me to develop the term, "threatened pre-eclampsia," to provide early warning signals of the impending development of the more serious symptoms. It has worked for me in heading off this particular toxemia of pregnancy and even pregnant women can very easily look for the signs and be aware that they should make some changes in their dietary patterns. The signals include:

1. Blood pressure increasing irreversibly one to two points weekly above the 120 mm. Hg. level for the systolic pressure.
2. Weight gain is rapid and exceeds two-thirds of a pound weekly.
3. Edema or swelling is slight but nevertheless apparent.

Avoid Excess Weight Gain but Eat Nutritionally

With pregnant patients, I begin with the nutritional approach at the first contact. As soon as they come under my care, I stress and outline the four basic food groups—fresh fruits and vegetables, protein selections from poultry, fish, and lean cuts of meat, whole grain breads and cereals, and dairy products. I review what they have been eating and drinking, and if there are inadequacies, I emphasize the foods that will provide missing vitamins and minerals. Vitamin and mineral supplementation is also used to fill in, if necessary. If the patient is extremely interested, I may suggest that a hair analysis be done just to see if the necessary complement of minerals is in the diet. If the ladies follow the basic plan and come in regularly for blood pressure and weight checkups, they should have few if any problems. Slippage does occur, however, because not all have the same willpower. I use the early warning system mentioned previously to alert me to potential problems. If I see the weight going up, I will immediately review what the patient is eating and determine where cutbacks can be made without impairing the nutritional intake. In all of this, the husband can be a positive influence in seeing that his wife eats the proper foods and obtains the proper supplementation, and I will enlist his aid if possible. This might occur, for example, if he accompanies his wife on an office visit. He will be eating, basically, the same foods as his wife, and if he is supportive and encouraging, her role is made that much easier. In the event that I cannot stem the rapid weight gain through these measures, as a more drastic event I might suggest that hospitalization be necessary to bring the weight situation under control. It is the lesser of two evils when compared to the life-threatening aspects of eclampsia and the treatment measures that have to be instituted if it occurs. The mere mention of the possibility of hospitalization has a salutory effect on patients who are not being careful about weight control.

The usual multivitamin-mineral formulation that I include in the diet plan has the following potencies:

vitamin A	10, 000 I.U.
vitamin C	100 mg.
vitamin D	400 I.U.
vitamin E	100 I.U.
vitamin B-1	10 mg.
vitamin B-2	10 mg.
vitamin B-6	10 mg.
vitamin B-12	10 mcg.
niacin	10 mg.
pantothenic acid	20 mg.
folic acid	100 mcg.
biotin	30 mcg.
PABA	30 mg.
calcium	375 mg.
magnesium	200 mg.
zinc	3 mg.

manganese	3 mg.
potassium	50 mg.
copper	500 mcg.
iodine	100 mcg.
iron	20 mg.

Blood and other tests may prompt me, depending on the findings, to recommend added amounts of particular nutritional factors.

The eating plan can follow this general outline with substitutions within the food groups to allow for variety:

milk	three or more cups daily
meat, fish, poultry	three servings daily, six to eight ounces each; use lean meats and include organ meats, such as liver, once a week; avoid processed or luncheon meats to minimize such factors as sodium nitrite
vegetables	two or more servings daily; use raw, lightly cooked, or steamed vegetables; at least one serving (one cup) should be dark green or dark yellow vegetable
fruit	two or three servings daily; use fresh fruit as often as possible; an apple, orange, or banana can be considered a single serving; one serving should be of a citrus fruit
eggs	one to two daily; recommend soft or poached
bread and cereal	three servings daily; eat whole grain, perferably whole wheat breads; eat oat or shredded wheat cereals and sprinkle with wheat germ, one serving is equal to one slice of bread or one-half cup of cereal; slicing banana on cereal can take care of two nutritional factors in one serving.
water and other beverages	six glasses daily; preferably use distilled water; avoid caffeine in colas, coffee; avoid fruit drinks with high sugar content.
salt	many new low-sodium foods are on the market that can aid in reducing salt consumption and avoid possible swelling problems; iodized salt can be used in the event there is a suspected deficiency of iodine that could cause goiter in child or in mother

By following this kind of diet and supplementation program, the pregnant woman is providing the foundation for averting eclampsia and other possible complications. Close and frank consultation with the attending physician or obstetrician is always advisable. Equally important a result or benefit from this program is that the fetus is being furnished with its nutritional needs.

In Chapter 1, I mentioned the female patient who had delivered two babies who died at very early ages of a neuromuscular disease. Subsequently, we altered her nutritional intake and she gave birth to a healthy baby girl.

Here are a few more cases from my files illustrating how important it is for the pregnant woman to pay close attention to what she eats and the other points mentioned in the preceding. A referral to my practice was a 23-year-old patient who experienced the pre-eclamptic condition and lost her baby. In that pregnancy she had been allowed an excessive weight gain and, obviously, had not been careful in what she ate. When she came to me she said that the eclamptic symptoms she had experienced had left her not only in a weakened condition but also depressed, as a result of losing the baby. Obviously, she and her husband had wanted a baby very much and I told her that before they tried again, we would have to make sure this time that she was in the best nutritional state possible. She was about five foot five inches and weighed 145 pounds. I wanted to get her weight down and we got her promise to eliminate every conceivable high-calorie food in her diet—soft drinks, donuts, ice cream, and candy and substitute more in the way of protein. It took about six months but we eventually brought her weight down to 125 pounds. I prescribed a multivitamin-mineral formulation and the chelated calcium-magnesium supplement to help her with some premenstrual tension problems. After this preparation I felt she and her husband were ready for another pregnancy. She did become pregnant and we paid close attention to and monitored her weight gain throughout the pregnancy. There were no problems and she was overjoyed when she gave birth to a healthy baby boy.

Another case was that of a 29-year-old patient who, previously, had gone through pre-eclampsia two times. While she delivered two babies successfully, she, too, did not want to suffer through the experience again. She came to me after hearing my name mentioned by a friend I had helped through a difficult pregnancy. She had a slightly elevated blood pressure that we brought under control through a combination of nutritional supplements, including extra vitamin C, vitamin E, lecithin, and magnesium. The program was built on a foundation of a sound diet that included, perhaps, a little more vegetables, fruit, and whole grain foods. Again, what was appropriate in her case might not work in another. After this regime I felt her blood pressure was in a manageable area and I said it was okay, as far as I was concerned, for her and her husband to try for another baby. They were successful and I continued my close monitoring of blood pressure, weight gain, and any swelling that might occur. Everything went smoothly and she gave birth to a baby girl without any of the mental and physical trauma she had experienced before with the preeclampsia. She was relieved and happy to know that the birthing process can be a satisfying and trouble-free experience.

Breast Conditions

There are two conditions of the female breast that, in my medical practice, can have a nutritional relationship. As always, I advise the female reader with any comparable problem to consult with her physician and not attempt self-diagnosis or treatment.

Swelling and Pain

A common condition affecting the breast is swelling. This is often associated with the premenstrual period and will occur three to five days prior to the onset of menstruation. The breasts can swell to the point where they become painful and tender. This premenstrual edema or swelling is connected, in my opinion, with salt (sodium chloride) retention in the tissues. To maintain the proper electrolytic balance in the cells, the body's defense mechanism is to cause an accumulation of fluid that, of course, leads to the swelling of tissues. According to my reasoning, it appears that estrogen, which initiates and guides the menstrual cycle, has an affinity for sodium chloride. In some women, then, we have an excess of estrogen causing an electrolytic imbalance and the retention of body fluids. Breast tissue, because of its anatomical configuration and location, can be particularly susceptible to producing discomfort and pain.

Reducing Salt Intake Can Help

The principal nutritional recommendation that I have for my patients experiencing the problem is that they reduce salt consumption. This means not only watching the use of table salt on foods but, in addition, being aware of its presence in processed foods and dressings as well. For example, foods with a high salt content can include dressings, sauces, canned foods, catsup, cheese, butter, peanut butter, meats, frozen vegetables, snack foods, greens like dandelion and mustard greens, spinach and kale, and turnips. Fortunately, some of these food products are being made available in low-sodium-content form to make avoidance easier. In addition, I note in the women's magazines that recipes now have accompanying information that includes sodium content. This helps those of you with the problem to keep closer track of your sodium intake.

An accompanying symptom in a number of cases where there is swelling of the breasts is severe headache. Brain tissue is susceptible to this same type of swelling phenomenon. The result is a headache. Again, the reduction of salt intake should prove helpful in relieving this symptom.

An interesting sidelight to these problems is that I have prescribed the vitamin B complex, which seems to increase the metabolism of estrogen in the liver. It is my belief that, through this reduction of estrogen in the liver, there is an accompanying reduction in sodium chloride and alleviation of the painful swelling and headaches.

Fibrocystic Breast Disease

There is a chronic and relatively common condition of the female breast in which multiple cysts form. The cysts are small, approximately the size of a pea, and several can group together to form a definitely palpable mass.

Pain and discomfort accompany the condition that is known as fibrocystic breast disease. It is important that a proper diagnosis be made that includes either biopsy or aspiration of the cyst. The purpose is to determine if the cyst is only that and not a malignant growth.

In the event that the discomfort or pain can no longer be tolerated, the cysts can be removed surgically, or they can be allowed to remain and be observed for any unusual changes. Females having such problems should, of course, report any changes in color, size, and other features to their physicians.

Nonoperative Approach Leads to Use of Vitamin A

My interest in developing a different treatment resulted from a patient I operated for a cystic mass in one breast. While the patient was recovering from the operation, we saw that the other breast started to develop the same kind of cystic mass. At the same time, I noted that the patient's skin was dry, her hands and feet were cold, and she complained of tiredness. I ordered a test that showed that she had a low-functioning thyroid. I prescribed thyroid extract to treat this particular problem and was astonished to see that the cysts in the breast cleared up. Subsequently, I have had good results in treating fibrocystic breast disease using thyroid extract when there is associated low-functioning thyroid.

From this case evolved a nutritional approach to this medical problem. I noticed that a number of my patients who had palpable masses indicative of cystic disease also had rough, dry breasts. While there was accompanying dry skin, tests did not point to a low-functioning thyroid. About this time I was using vitamin A to treat patients with sebaceous cysts of the skin and I was obtaining good results. It occurred to me that, perhaps, vitamin A might also be effective with cysts of the breast. I tried the treatment with a number of patients and it produced good results.

The symptoms that I look for to determine a vitamin A deficiency is if there is night blindness as in being unable to face the lights of oncoming cars. Or, it can be any sort of squinting to avoid the glare of bright light or sunlight. Some of these patients find it necessary to wear sunglasses almost continually when outdoors. In addition, there is a blood test that can be used to diagnose vitamin A deficiency.

Vitamin A and Breast Cysts

A typical patient was a 40-year-old woman who had a number of cysts in both breasts and her skin was quite dry. She complained of the discomfort and the appearance of her breasts that the cysts were causing. Mammography showed no malignancy and testing for thyroid function revealed no hypothyroidism. I began treating her with vitamin A. Once a week she was given 50,000 units of vitamin A by injection and she was also prescribed a formulation that provided an oral dosage of 10,000 units daily.

After the first few weeks, I reduced the injection dose to 25,000 units of vitamin A and after another few weeks eliminated it entirely. After that she was told to continue with the oral vitamin A at 10,000 units. It took approximately five months for the cysts to disappear entirely. While this may seem a long period of time, patients who elect to try the nutritional route prefer it to undergoing surgery.

A second case was that of a patient 32 years of age who came in with a history of sudden development of a mass in her right breast. Diagnostic tests confirmed it to be a cystic mass. No evidence of malignancy was found. I started the same course of treatment as in the first case and comparable results were obtained.

Again I wish to caution against self-treatment of any cystic mass with vitamin A without counsel from a physician.

Effect of Caffeine on Cystic Mastitis

Here is some interesting information for the heavy coffee drinkers among female readers. A paper, "Dietary Methylxanthines and Fibrocystic Breast Disease," by John P. Minton, M.D., which was given at a meeting of the International College of Surgeons, reviews the relationship of caffeine (methylxanthines) consumption to cystic mastitis. The study included 85 patients. Of the 45 patients who stayed away from coffee completely, 37 had "complete resolution" of the disease. Of 28 who cut their consumption, seven "resolved their disease," fourteen were improved, and seven remain unchanged. Of twelve patients who did not stop or cut down, nine remain unchanged, one improved, and two "resolved" the disease.

The results are a strong argument for females to reduce and, preferably, eliminate caffeine in whatever form from the daily diet.

Chapter 17

Diarrhea

Diarrhea can be a symptom of a wide range of medical problems. These include, but are not limited to, colitis, diverticulosis, amoebic dysentery, gastritis, gastroenteritis, and tumors. When accompanied by fever, loss of appetite, bloody stools, vomiting, loss of weight, and weakness, it is part of a more serious medical condition. Diarrhea, depending on its severity, can cause impaired absorption and loss of vitamins, minerals, sodium, potassium, and protein, all of which need to be replaced. When it lasts for more than a few days, dehydration and weight loss occur. Severe diarrhea is debilitating and requires more intense medical care.

What follows is not directed to the types of diarrhea with severe consequences.

I have had a number of patients come into the office with complaints of an intermittent type of diarrhea, usually resulting from a colitis or diverticulosis.

In colitis we find intermittent bouts of diarrhea or loose bowel movements, increased gas, abdominal pain with cramps, and some nausea. Diverticulosis is a condition in which there are small pockets or diverticuli of the colon. There may be alternating diarrhea and constipation, and abdominal pain and cramps in the lower left abdomen.

How to Restore Your Bacterial Balance and Eliminate Diarrhea with Acidophilus Bacillus

After diagnostic tests have confirmed what I am dealing with, I have obtained good results in treating the diarrhea in these cases by prescribing tablets or powder containing acidophilus bacillus. What I am attempting here is restoring the normal bacterial balance or flora of the large intestine to promote normal digestive processes.

The large intestine is the home of various bacterial and other microscopic forms of plant life that play a key role in good digestion. Bacterial concentration and variety are more intense in the large intestine than anywhere else in the entire gastrointestinal system. Approximately 100 million bacteria are present per ml. of intestinal content. In addition, while movement of food from the stomach to the end of the small intestine may take 30 to 90 minutes, passage in the colon may require one to seven days. Many foods not digested by the intestinal tract are broken down by this intense combination of bacteria and slower passage time in the colon.

Diarrhea can arise in the colon as a result of incomplete digestion taking place in the small intestine. For example, lactose, or milk sugar, is normally broken down in the small intestine and completely absorbed. However, if it reaches the large intestine in quantity it can precipitate diarrhea.

Antibiotics can also produce diarrhea. If I have patients referred to me by other physicians and there is a complaint of diarrhea, I check to see if possibly they have been treated with antiobiotics for infections. Similarly, if I have my own patients on antibiotics, I tell them to keep me informed if a diarrhea develops. Patients who have undergone surgery may be subjected to intensive antibiotic therapy and susceptible to an attack of diarrhea. Antibiotics do not discriminate and they destroy infectious bacteria, as well as the bacteria important for the proper functioning of the large intestine in the digestion and absorption of food.

Acidophilus baccilus helps restore the balance of the intestinal flora of the colon. In diverticulosis, for example, it is important that incompletely digested food not get lodged in the pockets or diverticuli and that intestinal bacteria do as efficient a job of digestion as possible. Otherwise, toxins can form in the pockets producing infections with more serious problems.

Another source of acidophilus baccilus that can be used is yogurt. I recommend the plain, unsweetened, and unflavored kind.

Diarrhea Attacks Cured

One of the cases of the milder type of diarrhea that I treated was that of a female patient, 49 years of age, who had a definite diverticulosis and alternating bouts of diarrhea and constipation. She reported that she had to be very careful in eating too much of high-fiber-type foods. Anyone with this condition should monitor their intake of high-fiber foods and be alert to note any association of a diarrheal condition with the foods. In the case of the patient, she reported that her husband had the same diarrheal condition. I prescribed a dosage of one or two tablets of acidophilus baccilus in the morning, in order to prepare their digestive tracts for whatever they were going to eat during the day. Within two weeks both wife and husband reported experiencing relief from the diarrhea. When this change occurred, I advised that they could eat normally without being overly concerned about the roughage in their diets. Because of possible loss of vitamins and minerals, I also prescribed a multivitamin-mineral combination formula for the wife and husband.

Another case was that of a woman, 45 years of age, with a diagnosed condition of diverticulosis. She too, I learned, had to be careful in avoiding foods that added too much roughage—whole grain cereals, raw vegetables, and various fruits. The resulting diarrhea, if she were not careful, could be quite severe for her. I prescribed the acidophilus tablets, and within ten days, the diarrhea slowed and finally stopped. After she resumed having normal bowel movements, I told her to try bran flakes in the event she saw a need for more fiber in her diet. She tolerated the bran flakes well and reported no further problems with the diarrhea.

To repeat, no severe diarrhea with the accompanying symptoms mentioned in the first paragraph should be treated lightly. Always consult with a medical doctor.

Dr. Daro's Guidelines for a Lifetime of Health and Well-Being

Chapter 18

Dr. Daro's 15 Cardinal Rules for Staying Healthy and Living Longer

Too many people eat and drink too much of the wrong foods and drinks simply because the foods and drinks are there. Hundreds of new foods and drinks are introduced each year. Unfortunately, not many are developed with the goal of providing us with sound nutritional benefits. In addition, too many food products are introduced with the objective of only providing a different and usually, sweeter taste.

It's not a bad idea to have a variety of choices but the emphasis in new foods has been in providing calories in the form of starch or sugar. For many of us it begins early in life with presweetened cereals and appetite-filling snacks. By the time adulthood is reached, it is difficult to switch to a diet that provides the essential nutrients that enable our bodies to manufacture the critically important amino acids, enzymes, and other raw materials that power our cells. This conditioning to the wrong foods is one reason why we have 60 million overweight people in the United States.

In the past few years a barrage of new food offerings has arrived on the market. These products include items like French onion-flavored dip, pineapple cheesecake cups, fruit punch-flavored cereals, and single-serving packets of artificial orange and lemon drink.

What does the dizzying array of food products tell us? It states that too often in reaching for something new to offer, many food manufacturers simply fall back on heavily sweetened products, drinks formulated with artificial flavors, and snack foods based on the use of artificial flavors. The inherent problem with food products of this kind is if they are consumed to the point where they replace needed food essentials.

Your Health Is Up to You

The real bottom line in this situation is you, the individual, health-conscious consumer who knows and understands what the essential nutrients are and makes sure that these are eaten first. All of the advertising and promotion in the world for empty-calorie foods is meaningless when you decide that you will not rely on snack foods, sugared cereals, and artificial drinks to meet your body's nutritional requirements. The decision to provide your body with vitamins, minerals, protein, carbohydrates, fiber, natural liquids, and fat in the right amount is yours. Out of the profusion of food offerings, you are the one who decides what to buy and eat and what to skip. When you decide to have an apple for dessert in place of a cream-filled eclair, you are doing your body a big favor and, I think, the nation's health bill.

As more and more people (and their numbers are increasing) make similar decisions that natural foods provide greater health benefits, food manufacturers will place fewer of the other foods on supermarket shelves. You don't have to write letters to congressmen protesting that this cereal or that fruit drink is bad for your health or that of your family. Instead, you just stop buying what you feel is not good for you and it will quickly and surely disappear from view.

Husbands, wives, single people, and even children who are interested in good nutrition and their health need to sort the real, genuine, and natural products out of the mountains of artificial foods. In this task you have the assistance of easy-to-read labels of the ingredients of various food products. Walk on by the displays of sweet, rich, and creamy desserts, cookies, and cakes. Become your own nutritional best friend. Treat your body kindly and it will render many years of good and faithful service. Load it up with junk and don't be surprised if you have to pay for it.

1. *Reduce Consumption of White Flour Foods.* Reduce or eliminate the amount you consume of pastries, breads, snacks, and other food products made with white flour. You ask, "What about enriched flour?" Enrichment is a stopgap solution to providing the consuming public with the proper nutrients. To have a manufacturing process strip away vital minerals and vitamins at one stage and then add them back at another flies in the face of logic. Obviously, also, only a partial restoration can and is made of the original nutrient content, and only those things are added back that scientists have up to this point in time identified as being required for human growth and maintenance. In other words we are being asked to wait for the signal to be given for the discovery that, yes, selenium, chromium, or another nutrient is okay before including it in our diets. The fact that some of these nutrients may have been consumed for thousands of years seemingly does not enter into the case. Until modern-day scientists have completed their research work, scientific groups and regulatory agencies withhold their approval of various nutrient materials. Before the advent of these groups, people ate foods in the natural state and lived, in many cases, to ripe old ages. Then, perhaps fortunately, there was no one around to warn against the consumption of something that had not been thoroughly researched beforehand. The vitamins and minerals were always there, we must remember. Nutritional scientists did not invent them. Somehow people obtained the benefits of these nutrient materials by consuming whole grains and cereals, unsprayed fruits and vegetables, and naturally fed livestock without the benefit of antibiotics and hormones.

Bake your own breads and cakes with unprocessed flour obtained from health food stores. Some supermarkets, also, are starting to stock natural flours.

One-hundred-percent whole wheat breads have always been available and in recent years they have become even more visible in food marts.

Don't assume that a dark bread is natural. Read the label. All too often you will see caramel coloring listed. Caramel is, of course, made by cooking sugar until it changes color. Real, natural flours do not have to be colored.

Another source of breads and other baked goods made from real flours are neighborhood bakeries. In the Chicago area, for example, there are a number of ethnic bakeries that make their breads and other baked goods with natural ingredients. If you have such bakeries where you live, this may be a solution to obtaining natural ingredients in baked goods. Many large bakeries, too, are now supplying supermarkets with baked goods made with natural ingredients. Perhaps the most satisfying option is to make your baked goods yourself using natural ingredients.

2. *Be Wary of Fad Diets.* Be wary of fad diets and weight-reducing products. Hardly a year goes by without one or two diet books high on the best seller list. Some of the diets advocated by the books are just variations of a basic, safe, 1000 to 1200 calorie balanced diet. However, some of the advice may be dangerous because the books emphasize one food or food groups. Simply put, they push unbalanced diets.

I want to point to one example to illustrate that care must be taken with any program for weight reduction that relies on a single product.

The Food and Drug Administration has issued requirements that very low-calorie protein diet products carry prominent warnings that their use as a total diet without medical supervision "may cause serious illness or death." Although the liquid protein diet fad is over, the FDA says some very low-calorie protein diet products are on the market and such fads tend to be revived.

Under the regulation, protein products deriving more than 50 percent of their calorie value from protein and represented for weight reduction must carry the statement:

> "—Warning—Very low calorie protein diets (below 400 calories per day) may cause serious illness or death. *Do not use for weight reduction in such diets without medical supervision.* Not for use by infants, children, pregnant, or nursing women."

Protein products designed to be used as a part of a total diet providing more than 400 calories per day, or as a food supplement, need not carry the warning but must state one of the following:

"—Notice—For weight reduction, use only as directed in the diet plan described herewith... Do not use in diets supplying less than 400 calories per day without medical supervision." (Manufacturers have the option of including a brief description of the diet plan with the label or informing consumers that the diet plan can be obtained by mail.)

"—Notice—Use this product as a food supplement only. Do not use for weight reduction."

The regulation requires that the statements appear "prominently and conspicuously on the principal display panel of the package label and any other labeling."

The regulation is the result of a government investigation in 1978 of deaths that were associated with the use of these products. By the end of 1977, the FDA had received 40 reports of such deaths—and more than 20 additional reports were received in 1978. A specially formed U.S. Public Health Service Protein Diet Task Force found that 17 of the deaths in otherwise healthy persons could be attributed directly to the diets. The unit concluded that protein products used as the principal or sole source of nourishment for rapid weight reduction may cause heart irregularities that may lead to death.

The FDA has repeatedly warned that *any* diet, high protein or otherwise, that provides less than 800 calories a day should be considered experimental and should be undertaken only with proper medical supervision.

The labeling requirements for protein diets do not apply to ordinary protein-rich foods such as meat or cottage cheese.

3. *Get Your Protein from Natural Sources.* Get your protein from natural sources and be sure to balance with carbohydrate and fat. Your natural sources include: milk, eggs, cheese, meat, and fish. Peanuts are a good source of protein; however, not all people have the digestive apparatus to handle them. As in all things, you need to sort out those foods that have proved themselves to be a source of distress. You have to learn to *be your own nutritionist.* For

example, while liver is a veritable storehouse of vitamins and minerals—chiefly iron and the B vitamins—it is not universally a favorite food. To obtain some of its benefits, you might try dessicated liver. All of the important foods are available in another form and if, for some reason, you can't adjust to them in their natural or regular form, then these alternate forms are there for you to try.

Protein is important as a source of eight amino acids that are essential for cell growth and maintenance. The foods containing the amino acids are said to have high nutritional value. The foods containing proteins of high value include: meat, fish, eggs, milk, and cheese. While beans, soybeans, peas, lentils, and cereals contain protein, they are of lesser value. Mixtures of the two types of protein-containing foods are more tasty and less expensive. Eating a wide variety of foods assures one of obtaining the most diverse supply of the amino acids and other necessary vitamins and minerals.

For daily meals to contain protein, a portion needs to be derived from animal sources. Cereal and vegetable foods combined with meat or fish improves the protein value of the meal. One way of doing this is to combine cereal with milk or cream, rice and fish, spaghetti and meat sauce, and vegetable stew with beef or lamb.

Body cells require protein for growth, repair, and maintenance. Protein also serves to make hemoglobin, which transports oxygen to cells and carries carbon dioxide away from the cells. Protein is the building block for antibodies that make up the immune system for fighting infection. Protein is also a source of energy.

4. *Keep Fat Consumption Moderate.* Keep the total amount of fat moderate in your daily meals and include mainly those foods that contain unsaturated fats.

Cooked fats add flavor and variety to foods. In addition, because fats digest slowly and delay hunger, they make foods and meals satisfying. But, as mentioned elsewhere, do not use snack foods too heavily because of their high-shortening content. They tend to kill the appetite for more important foods.

5. *Eat Fresh Vegetables.* Avoid the canned variety and stick with the fresh vegetables. There's too much salt used in canned vegetables. Because of this, you're not in charge of what's going into your body.

Frozen vegetables are a second choice, only if you can't buy the fresh ones.

But, in most places in the United States, you can always buy some fresh vegetables the year 'round. I've not been anywhere where fresh lettuce, for example, is not available. The same goes for many other vegetables—tomatoes, broccoli, carrots, cauliflower, etc. In essence, then, there is actually no reason to use canned or frozen vegetables when there is always some kind of fresh vegetable around.

As I pointed out in the beginning of this book, avoid overcooking. All that you do is leach out important minerals into the water and, at the same time, the heat destroys vitamins.

All of us do not like or can adjust to the taste of all vegetables. However, to try to obtain their nutritional benefits, give as many vegetables as possible a taste test. As the saying goes, "Try it, you might like it." Try not to reject some food or vegetable simply because you do not like the way it looks. The more that you try and learn to like, the greater will be the range of choice for having or selecting at least one fresh vegetable served with your meals. If one of your favorite vegetables is out of season or perhaps available only at high cost or in poor quality, then you can fall back on the other vegetables that you have tried and become familiar with.

6. *Eat Fresh Fruits.* The same suggestions apply to fruits as to vegetables.

Eat fresh fruits. Canned fruits are overwhelmingly sweetened. Fresh fruit—peaches, plums, nectarines, bananas, melons, apples, cherries, grapes, etc.— will provide you with all the sugar you need. In addition, the skins of many fruits supply you with valuable nutrients that are lost when they are peeled and packaged in jars or cans.

In addition, there's nothing more pleasurable than biting into a peach, for example, and tasting its own natural juices. This experience is never duplicated when you eat a canned peach that has been swimming in a heavy syrup.

Eating fresh fruit, such as an apple, is a lot more valuable for the health of your gums and teeth. The tearing action provides valuable exercise.

7. *Avoid Spicy Foods.* Avoid highly spiced foods. They can be irritating to the gastrointestinal tract and set the stage for inflammation and ulceration. Prepare foods with mild seasoning.

Too often in restaurants, seasoning is used in excess to cover up or disguise the taste of poor cuts of meat. The theory is that by stimulating the taste buds and the flow of saliva with sharp spices, the bland and tasteless cut of meat will pass through the mouth unnoticed. If you encounter food frequently prepared in this manner in the restaurants you visit, avoid these establishments. Your taste buds will become so accustomed to spices and seasonings that everything will start to taste bland if not similarly prepared. This overstimulation simply lays the groundwork for inflammation of the lining and tissues of the entire gastrointestinal tract. Ulcers and more serious consequences can result.

8. *Exercise—Do It!* Do it. Walk, swim, jog, bicycle, or do stretching exercise. Play tennis, volleyball, golf, racquetball, ping pong, or ride a stationary bicycle. Whatever the activity, do it regularly.

9. *Drink Natural Liquids.* Use the fresh and natural. Buy fresh orange or grapefruit juice or make it yourself. Don't use the artificial formulations that are usually identified as drinks rather than juices. Health food stores are good sources for a variety of fresh fruit drinks. The new blending machines are terrific for concocting new drink combinations.

Milk has a calming effect and is a good beverage before bedtime.

10. *Decaffeinated Coffee—If You Must.* If you need coffee, many decaffeinated brands are available. Tea, however, may be a better choice.

Tea in moderation is a soothing drink. Its tannic acid content can be neutralized to a degree by diluting with ample quantities of milk.

11. *Drink Distilled or Spring Water.* Water these days from our municipal sources is a suspect liquid. The chlorination and other chemical treatment turns ordinary water into a chemical formulation. Plenty of distilled and spring water is around to substitute for tap water.

12. *Avoid Soft Drinks.* Avoid soft drinks completely. If not possible, use only in moderation.

The caffeine and sugar are not designed to provide you with the essential nutrient to maintain your body physiology.

There are other thirst quenchers you can use like fruit juices, milk, and cold spring water.

An occasional beer is okay. Try to get one of the full-bodied, imported beers. The breweries in Germany and other countries, for example, are not as chemical oriented as here. Of late, we are seeing some of these imported beers taking a good share of the beer-drinking market. Guinness Stout, from Ireland, has actually been touted for its medicinal value because of its high mineral content.

A glass of wine now and then is satisfactory. It's more acceptable as a tranquilizer than whiskey. It's better than some of the complicated and addictive chemical formulae emanating from the drug companies.

13. *Don't Smoke.* No matter how low the tar and nicotine content in the newer cigarettes, you're far better off if you stay away from smoking. The number and kind of flavoring compounds is large and they are not identified. Who knows what their long term effect might be?

14. *Help Your Digestive Process by Chewing Well.* Chew and break up foods, especially meat, thoroughly. The smaller portions make the digestive process easier in your stomach and intestines. There is a safety factor involved, too, If you're eating meat, for example, smaller portions are less apt to get caught in the windpipe and if they are lodged there, they're easier to dislodge.

15. *Make Time for Relaxation.* In addition to the obvious benefits of sleep, we need to achieve states of relaxation other ways. One way to relax, obviously, is to avoid stress whether it's in the form of nerve-jangling music, entertainment, playing cards, long-distance driving, or another form.

Learn what relaxes you and indulge in this when you feel stress and nerves creeping up on you. Reading a book, going to a movie, taking a sauna bath, or swinging on a swing. Whatever. Find a relaxation technique or apparatus.

For many people this might be a hobby—fixing cars, amateur radio, astronomy, painting, canning vegetables, cooking, collecting stamps, or photography. Use it as often as necessary to relax.

Chapter 19

Open Up an Individual Health Account

My conviction in the benefits of nutritional therapy stems from seeing the dramatic improvements in the health and well-being of people I have treated and counseled. One of the most vivid changes I saw take place was in a physician colleague of mine. On one occasion I remember seeing him walking down the hall of the hospital where we both practiced. I noticed that he was walking slightly bent over, very slowly, and with short steps. While I had previously noticed somewhat of a slowing down in his physical actions, this particular day struck home when I saw the deterioration that had occurred. I walked over to him and inquired as to what was wrong. He replied that if he walked any faster, his angina would cause pain and distress. Up to this time I was really not aware that he had angina. He was about 65 years old at this time. I spoke briefly with him and mentioned the results I had obtained with vitamin E and suggested that he take 600 international units of the vitamin every day.

He accepted my counsel and began to take vitamin E in the dosage that I had recommended. I continued to see and talk with him at the hospital as we made our respective rounds to our patients. As time went by, it was astounding and naturally gratifying to see the change that occurred. Gradually, his stride started to lengthen and quicken. His posture became more erect. Within six months he regained his former strength and energy and reported to me that he was carrying out his medical duties without fatigue or the angina pain. This doctor expressed his appreciation to me more than once as we saw each other because he loved the practice of medicine and was able to continue seeing and treating patients. I was also pleased that he started to incorporate some of my nutritional ideas into his own practice and the treatment of patients.

In a sidelight to this story, this doctor asked his cardiologist about the value of vitamin E. My physician friend reported that the cardiologist scoffed at the idea of the use of vitamin E in cardiovascular problems. Interestingly, the cardiologist was also a friend of mine. One day when I met the cardiologist, he looked at me, threw his arms up into the air and exclaimed, "August Daro, what are you doing to yourself. Every time I see you, you seem to be getting younger." Immediately, I responded, "Vitamin E." Well, he appeared disbelieving and skeptical. I said, "Bill, keep your mind open. Try to learn things that are new."

About three weeks later, the doctor that I was treating with the vitamin E told me that the cardiologist called him and asked what dose of vitamin E he was taking. I chuckled and was pleased with the thought that I might be gaining another convert to the benefits of nutritional therapy.

In another sidelight to the story, I met the doctor that I had treated with vitamin E coming into the hotel where I was staying in Rome, Italy. At the time there was a general strike of workers going on in Italy and travelers were having to fend for themselves. This meant, for example, carrying and handling your own luggage. I was pleasantly surprised to see him entering the hotel with his wife, carrying luggage in both hands and, obviously, looking and feeling fit and well. When his wife saw me, she embraced me and thanked me for what I had done for her husband.

My Most Satisfying Years of Medical Practice

These past 20 years of my practice have been among the most satisfying of my entire medical life. As has been recorded in the preceding pages, I have been fortunate in being able to help a large number of people through nutritional means.

Throughout this phase of my medical practice, I have learned that many people could be helped simply and effectively by changing their dietary habits. Where there were medical problems that proved resistant to conventional medical therapy, it was gratifying to apply nutritional solutions and note that they produced results. In some cases, as with multiple sclerosis, while there was not a "cure" as such brought about, the patients still seemed to have held their own without any additional regression.

Nutritional therapy is at once a simple and complex method. It is simple because the nutrient materials, in general, are found in relative abundance in our food supplies. We do not have to wait for research scientists to discover, identify, or synthesize these materials. The nutrients are, and were always, there. What remained to be discovered were the roles they play in keeping our bodies going at an optimum level of performance. Nutritional therapy is somewhat complex in that knowing how much of the vitamins and minerals are necessary for each individual at each stage of life, and under various conditions of health and disease, is not yet an exact science. Because of this, anyone wishing to be helped through nutritional science should seek out an experienced and reputable practitioner in the field.

But, even before you consult with a nutritional therapist, why not try to establish the proper foundation by running an inventory of your dietary habits. Do you eat on a regular basis from the following list of basic foods:

1. fresh fruits
2. fresh vegetables
3. lightly cooked vegetables
4. meat
5. fish
6. dairy foods
7. water
8. fiber

9. whole grains in cereal and breads
10. unsaturated spreads or dressings

Are you eliminating or keeping at a minimum the consumption of:

1. coffee
2. tea
3. alcoholic drinks
4. soft drinks (especially those made from cola)
5. margarines and other spreads containing saturated fats
6. pies, cookies, pastries
7. any baked goods made from white flour
8. candy
9. sugar
10. heavily salted foods
11. overly cooked vegetables
12. fried foods

Are you getting enough physical activity on a regular basis?

Once you have established a sound dietary program, then you might consider a multivitamin-and-mineral preparation, just to be sure that you receive all of the essential nutrients.

From this foundation, you can consult with a nutritional expert for any specific problem with the expectation that his or her job in helping you will have been made substantially easier.

Whether you have a specific medical problem or not, it is still good philosophical and economic sense to place health in the first priority position. Today, the buzzword in so many spheres of living is "priority." What comes first? Place health in the first, or top, priority position. And, the beautiful part about such an objective is that it is an inexpensive investment and pays the largest dividends.

The talk all over is about IRAs, or Individual Retirement Accounts, and how it will assure a comfortable retirement.

Now is the time for you to set up an IHA, or Individual Health Account.

Here's what you have to invest:

a sound diet

exercise

essential vitamins and minerals

sufficient sleep for body repair and restoration

hobbies and interests different than the activities of work

moments of quiet, tranquility and peace

Here's what you will receive in the way of dividends:

a life that should provide you with the energy to fulfill your work obligations easily

a life that will make you an enjoyable companion

a life that will be interesting each day, week, month, and year

a *healthy* life

Nutritive Value of Foods in Calories

Dairy Products		Protein	Fat	Carbohydrate
cheese				
Cheddar	1 oz.	28	81	trace
cottage cheese				
small curd	½ cup	52	40	12
low-fat (2%)	½ cup	60	18	16
pasteurized process cheese				
American	1 oz.	24	81	trace
Swiss	1 oz.	28	63	4
milk				
fluid				
whole (3.3% fat)	1 cup	32	72	44
low-fat (2% fat)				
no milk solids added	1 cup	32	45	48
low fat (1%)				
no milk solids added	1 cup	32	27	48
non-fat (skim)				
no milk solids added	1 cup	32	trace	48
buttermilk	1 cup	32	18	48
chocolate milk, regular	1 cup	32	81	104
dried				
buttermilk	1 cup	164	63	236
nonfat instant	1 cup	96	trace	140
milk desserts				
ice cream				
regular (about 11% fat)	½ pt.	20	126	128
soft serve (frozen custard	½ pt.	28	207	152
ice milk (about 4.3% fat)	½ pt.	20	54	116
yogurt (from low-fat milk)				
fruit-flavored	4 oz.	20	13.5	84
plain	4 oz.	24	18	32
eggs				
raw				
whole, without shell	1 egg	24	54	4
white	1 egg	12	trace	trace
yolk	1 egg	12	54	trace
cooked				
poached	1 egg	24	54	4
fats, oils; related products				
butter	1 pat	trace	36	trace

Dairy Products		Protein	Fat	Carbohydrate
margarine				
regular	1 pat	trace	36	trace
oils				
corn	1 tbsp.	0	126	0
olive	1 tbsp.	0	126	0
safflower	1 tbsp.	0	126	0
salad dressings				
French				
regular	1 tbsp.	trace	54	12
low-calorie	1 tbsp.	trace	9	8
Italian				
regular	1 tbsp.	trace	81	4
low-calorie	1 tbsp.	trace	9	trace
mayonnaise	1 tbsp.	trace	99	trace
fish, meat, poultry				
fish sticks, breaded, cooked	1 oz.	20	27	8
salmon	3 oz.	68	45	0
shrimp				
canned meat	3 oz.	84	9	4
French fried	3 oz.	68	81	36
tuna, canned in oil	3 oz.	96	63	0
bacon	2 slices	16	72	trace
beef, cooked				
roast, lean	1.8 oz.	56	63	0
steak				
lean and fat	3 oz.	80	243	0
lean only	2 oz.	72	36	0
lamb, cooked				
chop, lean and fat	3.1 oz.	72	288	0
chop, lean only	2 oz.	64	54	0
liver, beef, fried	3 oz.	88	81	20
pork, fresh, cooked				
chop, lean and fat	2.7 oz.	76	225	0
chop, lean only	2 oz.	68	81	0
sausage				
bologna	1 slice	12	72	trace
frankfurter	1 link	28	135	4
poultry				
chicken				
breast, fried	2.8 oz.	104	45	4
drumstick	1.3 oz.	48	36	trace
turkey, roasted, skinless				
dark meat	3 oz.	104	63	0
light meat	3 oz.	112	27	0

Dairy Products		Protein	Fat	Carbohydrate
fruits				
apples	1 apple	trace	9	80
apricots				
raw	3 apricots	4	trace	56
dried, uncooked	½ cup	14	4.5	172
dried, cooked	½ cup	8	4.5	108
avocados, raw	1 avocado	20	333	52
banana	1 banana	4	trace	104
grapefruit				
pink or red	½ grapefruit	4	trace	52
white	½ grapefruit	4	trace	48
muskmelons				
canteloupe	½ melon	8	trace	80
honey dew	½ melon	4	trace	44
oranges				
whole	1 orange	4	trace	64
peaches, raw	1 peach	4	trace	40
pears, raw, Bartlett	1 pear	4	9	100
prunes, uncooked	5 prunes	4	trace	116
grain products				
bagel				
egg	1 bagel	24	28	112
breads				
French, enriched	1 slice	12	9	76
Italian, enriched	1 slice	12	trace	68
rye, American, light	1 slice	8	trace	52
white, enriched	1 slice	8	9	48
whole wheat	1 slice	12	9	48
breakfast cereals				
hot-type, cooked				
oatmeal	1 cup	20	18	92
ready-to-eat				
bran flakes (40%)	1 cup	16	9	112
corn flakes, plain	1 cup	8	trace	84
rice, puffed, plain	1 cup	4	trace	52
wheat flakes	1 cup	12	trace	96
wheat, shredded	1 biscuit	8	9	80
cakes				
devils' food, chocolate icing	1 cupcake	8	36	80
Boston cream pie	1 slice	12	54	136
fruitcake, dark	1 slice	4	18	36
pound	1 slice	8	90	64

Dairy Products		Protein	Fat	Carbohydrate
cookies				
brownies with nuts	1 brownie	4	36	52
chocolate chip	2 cookies	4	40	58
crackers				
graham	2 crackers	4	9	40
saltines	4 crackers	4	9	32
Danish pastry				
round piece	1 pastry	20	135	120
donut	1 donut	4	45	52
macaroni, enriched, cooked				
tender stage, hot	1 cup	20	9	128
macaroni (enriched) & cheese				
canned	1 cup	36	90	104
from home recipe	1 cup	68	198	160
noodles (egg) enriched				
cooked	1 cup	28	18	148
pancakes, buckwheat	1 cake	8	18	24
pies				
apple	1 slice	12	135	204
pumpkin	1 slice	20	135	128
pizza	1 slice	24	36	88
popcorn, popped				
plain	1 cup	4	trace	20
with oil and salt	1 cup	4	18	20
rice, white, enriched				
instant, cooked, hot	1 cup	16	trace	160
long-grain, cooked, hot	1 cup	16	trace	200
spaghetti				
tender stage, hot	1 cup	20	9	128
waffles				
from home recipe	1 waffle	28	63	112
from mix, egg, & milk added	1 waffle	28	72	108
legumes (dry), nuts, seeds				
beans, dry				
lima, cooked, drained	1 cup	64	9	196
cashews, roasted in oil	½ cup	48	288	80
peanuts, roasted in oil	½ cup	74	324	54
peanut butter	1 tbsp.	16	72	12
sunflower seeds	½ cup	70	310	58

Dairy Products		Protein	Fat	Carbohydrate
sugars & sweets				
candy				
chocolate				
milk, plain	1 oz.	8	81	64
honey, strained or extracted	1 tbsp.	trace	0	68
sugars				
white, granulated	1 tbsp.	0	0	48
vegetables				
asparagus				
spears, raw	4 spears	4	trace	8
beans				
green, cooked, drained	½ cup	4	trace	14
broccoli, raw	1 stalk	24	9	32
cabbage				
cooked, drained	1 cup	8	trace	24
carrots, raw	1 carrot	4	trace	28
collards, raw	1 cup	28	9	40
corn, sweet				
raw, cooked, drained	1 ear	8	9	64
lettuce, raw				
crisphead (such as iceberg)	1 cup	trace	trace	8
onions, raw	½ cup	4	trace	20
peas, green				
canned	½ cup	16	4.5	58
potatoes				
baked	1 potato	16	trace	132
French fried	10 strips	8	63	72
mashed, milk added	1 cup	16	18	108
potato chips	10 chips	4	72	40
spinach, cooked, drained	1 cup	20	9	24
squash, cooked				
summer, drained	1 cup	8	trace	28
winter, baked	1 cup	16	9	128
tomatoes, raw	1 tomato	4	trace	24
miscellaneous items				
soups, prepared with equal amounts of water				
beef broth	1 cup	20	0	12
minestrone	1 cup	20	27	56
tomato	1 cup	8	27	64
vegetable	1 cup	8	18	52

Index

T

U

V